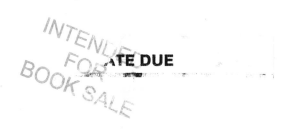

Yogilates®

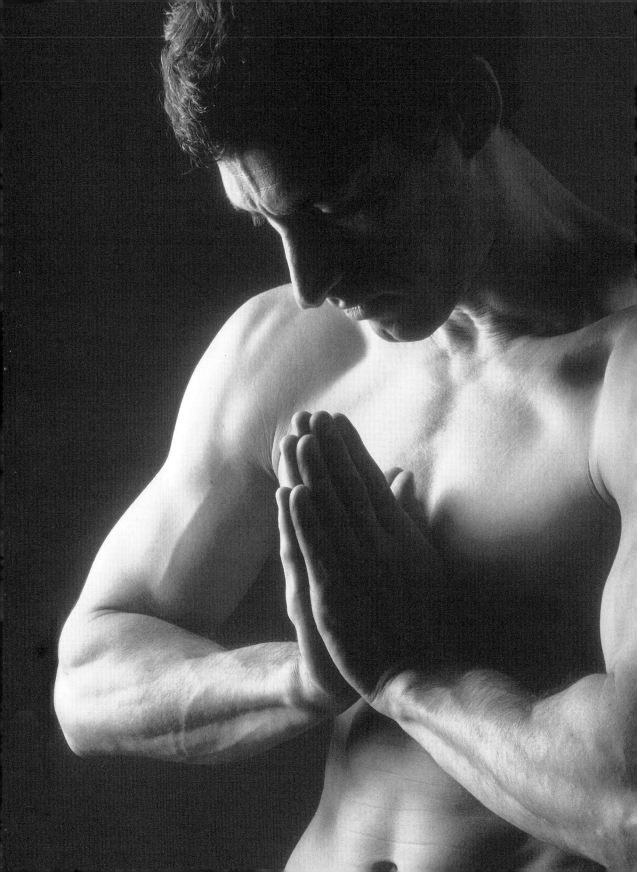

Yogilates®

Integrating Yoga and Pilates for Complete Fitness, Strength, and Flexibility

Jonathan Urla

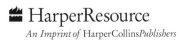
HarperResource
An Imprint of HarperCollins*Publishers*

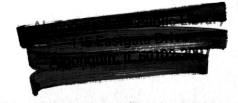

The information in this book has been carefully researched, and all efforts have been made to ensure accuracy. The author and the publisher assume no responsibility for any injuries suffered or damages or losses incurred during or as a result of following the exercise program in this book. All of the procedures, poses, and postures should be carefully studied and clearly understood before they are attempted at home. Always consult your physician or qualified medical professional before beginning this or any exercise program.

HarperCollins books may be purchased for educational, business, or sales promotional use. For information please write: Special Markets Department, HarperCollins Publishers Inc., 10 East 53rd Street, New York, NY 10022.

Yogilates is a trademark of Jonathan Urla and used with his permission.

FIRST EDITION

Designed by Ralph Fowler
Photographs by Kit Kittles
Illustrations copyright © by Nenad Jakesevic

Printed on acid-free paper

Library of Congress Cataloging-in-Publication Data has been applied for.
ISBN 0-06-001026-6

02   03   04   05   06   WBC/RRD   10   9   8   7   6   5   4   3   2   1

To Natalie

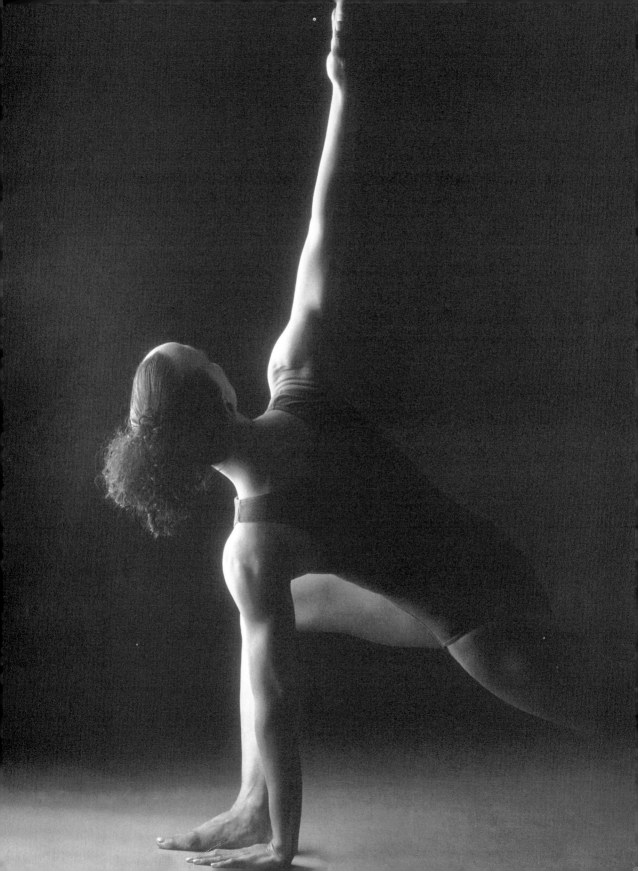

Contents

Acknowledgments

I would like to thank everyone who has helped and supported me in the writing of this book. It all began with finding the best literary agent in New York, Joy Tutela. Her encouragement, patience, and wisdom guided me whenever things got rough. I am also very grateful to my editor, Harriet Bell, and everyone at HarperCollins for their invaluable assistance and for having the faith to grant me the freedom to create the best book I could. I want to also thank my photographer, Kit Kittles, for his incredible eye, my illustrator, Nehad Jakesevic and my fabulous models, Patricia Levy and Judy Tyrus.

For their professional support and encouragement, I want to thank the Group Exercise Directors at New York Sports Clubs, Equinox Fitness Clubs, and Sports Club/LA. Special thanks also go out to Phoebe Higgins, Peter Roel, Bob Liekens, Power Pilates, and all my fellow yogis, especially Forest Gamble.

A very warm thank you to Claire Tornay, Gail Gittelson, and Linda Rossi as friends extraordinaire.

And big thanks to my brother Paul, and to my family who showed me faith and love all the time.

Yogilates®

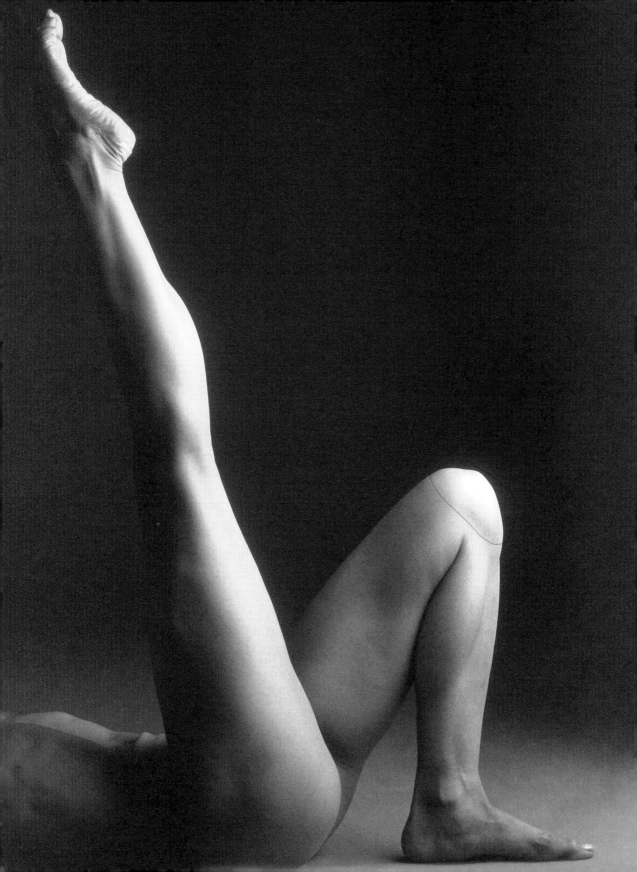

Introduction

Everyone wants a better body, a healthier, more toned, and more flexible body. For the longest time, I was convinced that the only way to transform my body, and those of my clients, was through intense training in the gym with weights and machines. A chiseled-looking body was relatively easy to attain this way. Eventually, however, I began to question the overall benefit of these workout routines. I was stronger than I ever had been, but my muscles were bulky and I had lost much of my natural agility, flexibility, and coordination. I noticed that my athletic performance in sports such as swimming, basketball, and tennis was actually hampered by my overdeveloped muscles. Most troubling of all, despite the fact that I stretched more than most people, I was more prone to injuries. I trained regularly and with good form, but my body was often achy, sore, and tight, making simple actions like bending over or reaching behind myself difficult. I realized that my harder and longer workouts were not giving me all the benefits that a truly complete fitness regimen should give. These dissatisfying results were not due to any particular exercises, weight lifting, or running; rather, by limiting my training to this conventional program, I felt I was neglecting other important areas of fitness. My body and my mind told me that I had had enough and I needed to reassess my regimen.

What happened to me is not uncommon. Many people lose sight of the ultimate purpose of exercise, which is to improve overall health and fitness. They become lost in the mindless patterns of the gym and habitually grind out set after set in strainful workouts. While it's important to build strength and increase muscle tone, that is simply not enough. Having overly developed leg muscles won't help you stretch up on your toes to reach for a box of cereal on the top shelf, nor will they help you regain your balance when you lose your footing. Likewise, having large shoulders is a hindrance when you have to reach down to retrieve a document from under the desk. A human body is meant for all kinds of movements, with overall performance measured in more than just pounds lifted or miles traveled.

What does it mean to be really fit? For me, I wanted to be more than just strong. I wanted to be agile, flexible, coordinated, and to have good balance—qualities of movement I associate with my youth when I was dancing and playing sports. But, these physical qualities are not just important in sports—they make everyday activities easier too. Being fit also means being less prone to injury, and having more energy to face life's chal-

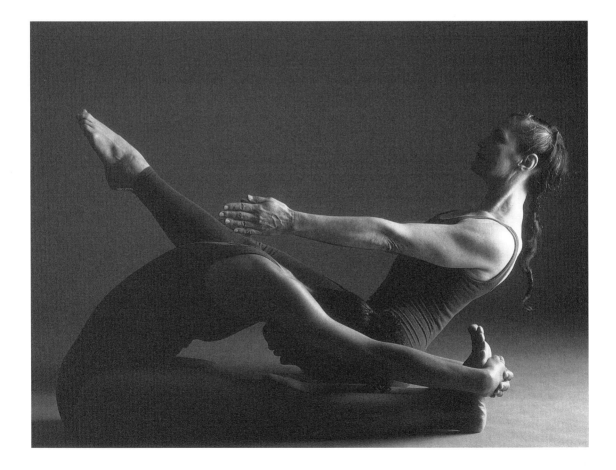

lenges. I realized that what I really wanted was a regimen that would add more freedom and skill to my movements without increasing the wear and tear on my body.

To do this, I realized my exercise program had to be multidimensional, incorporating a variety of skills, and it had to make me "functionally fit" for the long haul. All facets of fitness had to be addressed, including strength, flexibility, alignment, coordination, balance, and endurance. Moreover, strength must be measured not just in pure power, which can be abrupt or awkward, but in terms of stability and control. Likewise, flexibility should not be defined simply as loose muscles and joints, which are easily strained, but rather as moving fluidly through an expanded range of motion. Even the concept of balance needs to evolve to one of having dynamic poise and a sense of symmetry in space. Recently, new exercises have been developed that deal with different areas of functional fitness, from utilizing a physioball to improve awareness of alignment and balance to changing the speed of motion in resistance exercises. But, after exploring these ideas, and many others, I was still convinced that conventional methods would not provide me with a system of exercise that integrated all the elements of fitness for optimal health and longevity. Ultimately, I knew this would be a challenge for my mind as well as my body.

Yoga

The search for a more ideal system of training the mind and body for complete fitness first lead me to the ancient practice of yoga. As a dancer, I learned early on the value of using the postures and breathing of hatha yoga to enhance my flexibility. Hatha yoga is the physical practice of yoga that involves moving in and out of different positions called "asanas." There are hundreds of these exercises, their origins dating back some 5,000 years, to ancient India. The practice also involves breathing and meditative exercises, and is linked to other health and ethical practices of yoga through the "yoga sutras." Currently, there are many different styles of hatha yoga, including Astanga, Iyengar, Sivananda, Bikram, Kripalu, Vinyasa, etc. Ultimately, the practice of hatha yoga is meant to challenge and inspire you to greater physical, mental, and spiritual heights.

For me, there are four great benefits to practicing hatha yoga. By teaching you to exercise at a slower, more mindful pace, yoga helps develop greater inner awareness of yourself. Yoga also gets you to focus on your breathing, which helps your cardiopulmonary system as well as enhancing your efforts in flexibility and strength exercises. Learning the postures, one explores a wide variety of positions and movements, which develops greater skill and confidence in your mind and body. And last, but not least, yoga teaches you to relax your mind and body as a vital element of your practice.

In this fast-paced, constantly moving world, practicing yoga allows me time to stop and just be aware of where I am and how I feel. It is a time to be one with my body, and let go of all the distractions and worries of the outside world. Holding an asana like Warrior One, with my legs stretched in a lunge and my arms reaching up, I feel grounded and free at the same time. I can sense my body acting as a conduit between the earth and the sky, and feel my breath flowing with this sacred energy.

There are, however, some hatha yoga postures that can be risky and unwise for many people to practice. While not difficult for some, performing headstands, doing full back-bends, and even crossing the legs too much can strain the neck, spine, and knees. I've also found that a typical hatha yoga class allows for little time to warm up the body with preparatory movements and stretches. Performing the Sun Salutation series with its full-forward bends, lunges, plank positions, and so on early in the routine is difficult for most people, myself included. I wanted to experiment with the traditional sequences and wondered if a more user-friendly approach to the postures could be developed. Neverthless, I knew in my heart that with hatha yoga I had found an expansive, wise, and inspirational self-sufficient system of training the mind and body for better health.

Pilates

Pilates (pronounced puh-la-tees) is a method of exercise named after European fitness guru, Joseph H. Pilates. Born in Germany in 1880, Joseph early on devoted himself to fitness and became skilled at many sports, including gymnastics, diving, skiing, and boxing. As a young man, he traveled to England and worked as a circus performer and boxer. During World War I he was interned on the Isle of Man with other prisoners of war and took it upon himself to help rehabilitate the injured and sick and generally to boost their morale. Pilates returned home a war hero, but he soon became disenchanted with his new assignment of training members of the German military. He decided to emigrate to the United States, where he and his wife, Clara, opened an exercise studio in New York City in 1926. An ingenious inventor as well as a physical trainer, he created machines and various pieces of equipment, most notably the Universal Reformer. But his original technique was based on his matwork, or floor exercises, which use just the body and gravity for resistance to develop superior strength and flexibility. His studio attracted many

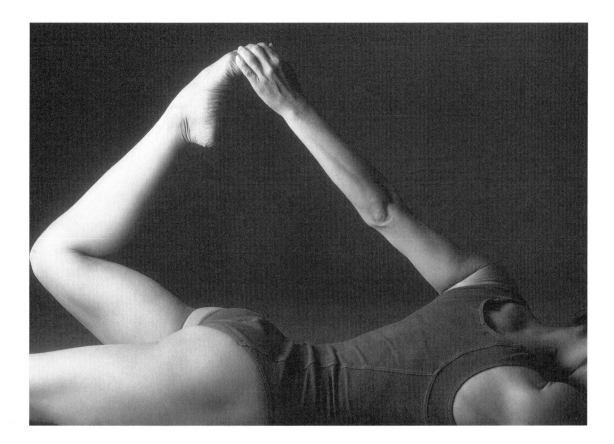

famous dancers and performers who needed to rehabilitate from injuries. Ballet master George Balanchine and modern-dance pioneer Martha Graham were among his many students.   78

Since Pilates' death in 1968, his technique has evolved under the various master instructors who teach his highly specific methods, many of whom are former dancers or physical therapists. What remains at the heart of Pilates technique is the development of powerful strength in the abdominals, spinal flexibility, and precise alignment of the body. Dancers and athletes love Pilates because it develops core strength and adds stability and control to their movements. Pilates instructors also emphasize a natural rhythm to the exercises, teaching students to connect the movements in a fluid and graceful manner. This requires coordination and concentration and translates to more efficient biomechanics and greater safety during exercise.

By teaching me to generate power from my core and maintain proper alignment, Pilates training helped me find my center. Although I stopped lifting weights, I became a stronger swimmer, runner, and dancer because I was utilizing deep torso muscles (my "powerhouse") for greater strength and was moving more efficiently and with better control. Nevertheless, I found that there were some Pilates exercises that overstressed certain areas of the body, particularly the neck. Moreover, I yearned to include stretches and movements in my workouts that were considered outside the strict vocabulary of traditional Pilates. Yet, as with yoga, I knew that Pilates technique was a gift and that its foundation was sound and true. The seeds of my future lifelong devotion had now been planted together. Mixed with the soil of current knowledge from exercise science and my own intuition, it was only a matter of time before it would all come to fruition.

Yogilates

On one particular day, I went to a yoga class right after a Pilates session. Despite the advanced level of the class, I found that the Sun Salutations and positions were much easier to achieve, and there was none of the back and leg discomfort I often felt before I warmed up. I also noticed I was able to stay better aligned in my postures and was using my core muscles for support, which immediately aided my practice.

Similarly, on another day when I reversed the order of my workouts and went to my Pilates session after a yoga class, I was able to relax and breathe more easily during the exercises, using the skills I had developed through my hatha yoga practice. It quickly became apparent that when I allowed each discipline to influence the other, there was a synergistic effect. By studying and practicing both, my body was feeling the best it had in 20 years! It was as if a lightbulb went on in my mind and body at the same time! While yoga generates awareness, endurance, flexibility and versatility from the various postures, Pilates matwork creates real core strength, precise alignment, and muscular coordination throughout your range of motion.

It was obvious to me that for optimal fitness, yoga and Pilates belonged together. Unfortunately, practicing both full regimens at the same time is not very practical for most people and could easily lead to overtraining. Yogilates was born from my desire to create an accessible and effective regimen that contained the best of both techniques and would be ideal for everyone, whether they had done yoga, Pilates, both, or neither. Beginning with basic functional and awareness skills, I want to help people grasp the essential principles of how to breathe correctly, engage the core muscles, and maintain postural alignment—the physical roots of yoga and Pilates techniques. My goal was to create time-efficient, balanced, and flowing routines that addressed all the areas of mind/body fitness, and that promoted the integration of the principles from both hatha yoga and Pilates. Many of the advanced exercises from each discipline are not presented here, as those experts who can do them don't need this book. However, as yoga and Pilates purists will agree, you don't have to be able to sit in full Lotus position or perform the Pilates Hundred with your legs 6 inches off the floor to successfully get all the benefits that yoga and Pilates have to offer.

Learning Yogilates will help you to focus with more clarity and give you a flatter tummy. It will teach you to sit and stand with better alignment and help you lose excess weight. Ultimately, it is designed to improve your overall health and fitness and gives you a versatile practice you can enjoy doing for the rest and best of your life. With the Yogilates Essential Awareness Exercises and routines for beginner to advanced, you can develop at your own pace and still be confident in the transformational power of your practice. To complete your fitness program you need to include regular cardiovascular activity along with your Yogilates routine, as recommended in the last chapter.

As you will see, the philosophy of Yogilates calls for you to integrate spirit and function in everything you do, and to never settle for less than your potential. Trust in yourself and listen to the inherent wisdom of your body. Yogilates is always about being good to yourself and appreciating the natural gifts you were born with. I hope you see Yogilates as one of the many positive things you have chosen to do for yourself as you journey toward a healthier, happier, and longer life.

Namaste.

Enjoy!

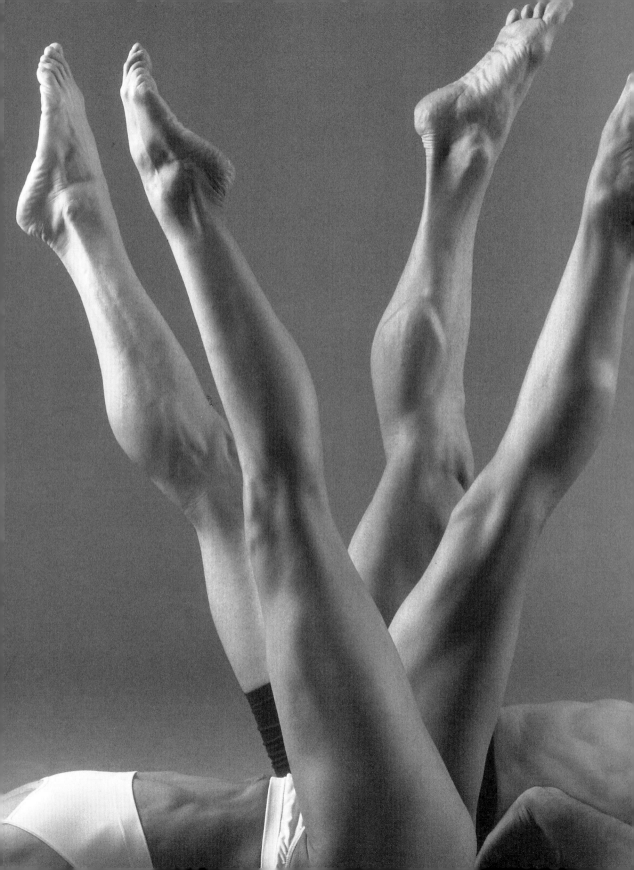

Chapter One

The Yogilates Philosophy

[Contrology] develops not only the muscles of the body, suppleness
of the limbs, and functioning of the vital organs and endocrine
glands; it also clarifies the mind and develops the will.
—J. H. Pilates

Asanas have been evolved over the centuries so as to exercise
every muscle, nerve and gland in the body.... But their real
importance lies in the way they train and discipline the mind.
—B. K. S. Iyengar

It is important to remember that, despite all the pictures of yoga and Pilates practitioners doing fantastic positions and movements with their bodies, it is the development of the mind that is most critical. This intangible aspect of our being, the way we think, ultimately shapes the development of our physical and spiritual self. Everyone starts out with primary instincts and a certain amount of raw talent. But your perception of yourself and your learned interests create reactions and physical habits that will really shape your body and greatly influence your overall well-being. Both yoga and Pilates were created with the belief that through disciplined practice, one cannot only develop tremendous physical skills and improve health, but can also transform oneself mentally and spiritually to a higher plane. Joseph Pilates first became famous not as a physical trainer, but as a volunteer nurse and morale leader for the sick and wounded in a World War I prisoner-of-war camp. The yoga master Krishnamacharya, who helped establish the Mysore hatha yoga schools in India, likewise felt that it was not the regimen of hatha yoga that was so important as its compassionate application to restore health and wellness to his students.

Most Westerners oversimplify their understanding of Eastern philosophy to the precept that the mind ultimately controls the body. But the notions of control and discipline both have negative connotations in Western culture and require further interpretation. The disciplined mind is sought after by practitioners for two reasons: First, it can identify and focus on difficult problems and improve skills. Simply put, if you focus on what you are doing as you practice, you are acting out your discipline. Second, the disciplined mind is valued because it protects the practitioner from inner chaos. Inattention and distraction are burdens on the mind and weaken the spirit. Controlling one's inner space leads to clarity of mind and freedom from stress, and ultimately to greater energy for living.

It would seem that establishing discipline in mind and body would be the first step toward superior fitness, but before discipline one must have commitment. That is why your spirit, that which drives you, must be there along with the science of the mind and body. For this, one must look to the heart. Ask yourself what you want from a fitness program and how that is related to your goals of everyday life. Do you see exercise as a golden opportunity to learn and enhance your skills, just as you would approach a career or new experience? Or do you see it more as a duty or a chore? The more your attitudes toward exercise are related to your everyday attitudes about how you want to lead your life, your own personal philosophy, the stronger will be your commitment to fitness. In this way, exercise is never a chore but a desire, even a passion, for experiencing life to its fullest.

The following philosophical guidance and wisdom I have learned from my elders. I share it so as to help you prepare mentally and spiritually to get the most from your Yogilates practice.

The True Self

I do not need to pretend that I am anyone other than
myself. I do not need to feel insecure about my perceptions.
The self-cultivation that I undertake is to perfect who I am,
not to become someone other than who I am.

—Deng Ming-Dao

As you prepare to begin practicing Yogilates, be aware of all the things you are bringing with you. Your body, of course, but also the way you think about your body. Maybe you see your body as run-down or old. Perhaps you see yourself as uncoordinated or clumsy. Maybe you just want it to change or to look like someone else's body. You need to be aware of your perceptions of your body and to see if you have negative ideas about it. We know that poor self-image, low confidence, and feelings of fear or shame have equally negative physical effects on our health and performance. You must be an *alchemist for the mind* and work to restructure negative thoughts into positive ones.

Realize that these negative ideas are not your true natural self. Your true self is the miracle of life that expresses itself through your body and spirit every day. Tell yourself that you are capable, and able to adapt and learn no matter what your age or condition. One way to appreciate your body more is to think of all that it does for you automatically. The autonomous systems of the body regulate your temperature, your organs, your digestive system, your senses, and so on. No matter what your body has been through, it is still here and performing miracles that machines will never be able to completely duplicate. Your true self is you and the life energy (called "prana" in yoga) that courses through your body with the air you breathe all the time. Everyone has this same life energy, and it is what joins us all in the potential for physical, mental, and spiritual well-being.

One of the things you will be asked to practice in Yogilates is simply to sit and follow your breath. So right now, close your eyes and start to breathe deeply through your nose. With each exhale visualize blowing out any worries, doubts, or fears. Clean out the negative perceptions of your body and abilities and breathe in pure oxygen and nurturing affection for your body. Just be clear and still and open to the possibilities that may arise from your practice. See your true natural self, a wonderfully curious being with a boundless store of courage, faith, and potential for growth.

The Process = the Goal

To live for some future goal is shallow. It's the sides
of the mountain that sustain life, not the top.

—Robert M. Pirsig, *Zen and the Art of Motorcycle Maintenance*

It is possible to use this book with the sole intention to achieve the postures and exercises of Yogilates. But the quality of your results will suffer greatly if you strive for the outcome without paying attention to the process of how you achieve it. Both yoga and Pilates call for a great deal of flexibility, not only in the body but also in the mind. They require you to let go of preconceived expectations or comparisons to others, as that will

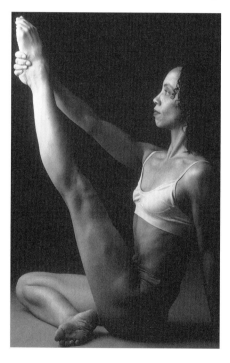

only lead to frustration. Every day I see people in classes who get down on themselves because they can't do a pose the way they think they should. They struggle rather than reach for more props, or hang out after class complaining to others of their shortcomings. They could have been having a wonderful class, moving synchronously with their breath and the other students, and then, by engaging in negative thinking about themselves, they completely stopped the flow of their workout and denied its benefits.

Real growth happens only when we let go of analytical thinking and limited goals and instead allow ourselves to be in the magic of the moment. Every moment of practice is an opportunity for greater awareness. In the beginning, you will learn to be a student again as you study "how" to do the exercises. As you progress, the process will become more experiential as you shift your attention to "what" you are doing. Learn to be present in your thinking and to appreciate the simple fact that you are breathing, moving, and enjoying the

real beauty of your practice. The truth is that there need never be another goal for Yogilates other than to listen to your body and express yourself physically every day as eloquently as you can. This makes every moment you practice a successful one. You cannot know exactly how long it will take to master certain skills of Yogilates, but you can know exactly how long it takes to master the *process* of learning those skills. Simply be open to communication with your body, and the moment has begun!

The Art of Practice

Practice your exercises diligently with the fixed and unalterable determination that you will permit nothing else to sway you from keeping faith with yourself.

—J.H. Pilates

The qualities demanded from an aspirant are discipline, faith, tenacity and perseverance to practice regularly without interruption.

—B.K.S. Iyengar

A commitment to regular practice is essential to master any discipline. The reason the masters wanted people to practice faithfully is because they knew that the greatest rewards come to those who are the most persistent and patient. The beginning will be the hardest time as you try to knock out a chunk of minutes from your normal schedule for practice time. For some people, exercising on their own allows greater freedom to practice whenever they can. For others, going to a class works best because they feel a commitment to a set time, place, and other like-minded individuals. However you begin, focus on getting your consistency up to 5 or 6 days a week. Soon, your mind and body will have become happily addicted to the stretching, relaxing, and energizing doses of Yogilates, and your yoga mat will become as familiar to you as your bed.

After the commitment to practice Yogilates regularly is established, the next stage is to absorb the technique. Someone once said that the secret to life is in the details. The same can be said of the art of practicing Yogilates! I remember a study done of different training techniques used by voice teachers in relation to the success of their students. An interesting fact was that the more successful teachers all had highly specific verbal and visual cues for what they wanted from the voice. For example, instead of just telling a student to open his mouth wide and relax the jaw, they might have asked the student to imagine his mouth as a bell and to feel the timbre resonating from all around the skull. According to Shirley Emmons, coauthor of *Power Performance for Singers,* utilizing creative visualization is not eccentric, but is firmly rooted in the science of training the mind and the body for optimal performance. According to theory, the brain is divided into two hemispheres, with one side handling the cognitive functions and the other absorbed with creativity and intuition. Performance results are most successful when you incorporate work for both hemispheres into your practice.

In Yogilates training, the precise alignment instructions will challenge the left side of your brain, while the sensory and creative imagery will stimulate the right side. This "whole-mind integration" is a key part of mastering Yogilates technique and requires attention and focus. Through mindful repetition, the details of the technique will be absorbed into your own muscle memory. Then, without much conscious effort, a single word or image will spontaneously create good form. You will be able to stop thinking so hard and observe yourself flowing harmoniously with your body and your breath. But there is no shortcut to this heightened awareness. It happens only after years of study and mindful practice. Do not count the days or look at a calendar, for that will only make it take longer. The effort may seem great, but it is only as much as it takes to practice today. If you are faithful to your practice, you will be rewarded.

Better Health and Enjoyment Through Moderation

Elegant sufficiency

—Romana Krysanowska

One of the hardest concepts to accept in our society is the notion of moderation. In Eastern philosophies, moderation has deep roots, as in the yoga concepts of *aparigraha,* meaning greedlessness, and *samtosha,* meaning contentment. The Tao philosophy refers to it simply as "nonexcessiveness" and it is equated with balance and longevity. In Western culture, as late as the early 1900s, there used to be the notion of one's "daily constitutional" or "setting-up exercise," which was usually a brisk walk outside and some light calisthenics. This was back in the day when a healthy lifestyle meant not exerting yourself too much and moderation was seen as a sign of good upbringing. Today, however, there is no holding back. Judging by our commercial culture, you would think that everything about sports or fitness these days has to be "extreme" to be really worth anything. Now most young people equate moderation with a lack of effort and boredom.

The truth is that a sense of moderation does not mean that the challenge is any less or that the practice is less exciting. In Yogilates, it means staying in the middle, between the two extremes of too little or too much. Think about the last time you felt you had "just enough" of something, whether it was a food or the pleasure of someone's company. You know the feeling, where one more bite or one more minute can quickly change a perfect

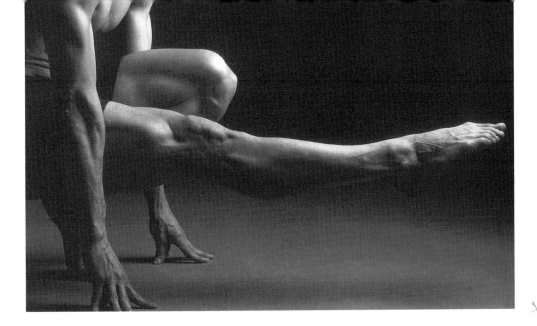

experience to regret. In terms of exercise, it means looking for satiation from your work-out rather than gratification. Joe Pilates understood early on that quality was far more important than quantity and specifically limited the number of repetitions for each of his exercises. His protégée, Romana Krysanowska, has a succinct and appealing phrase for this philosophy of holding back: elegant sufficiency.

You will find that Yogilates routines contain a reasonable amount of exercises to be performed at a moderate speed for a limited number of repetitions. In this way, you will avoid the common pitfalls of working out obsessively, including burnout, injury, and stress. The great truth is that not only is it healthier for you physically, mentally, and spiritually to work at an even pace, but you can actually achieve more with less. Optimal results are achieved only with a balance between the variety of exercises, the time expended, and the energy that is required to do them. Yogilates, like life, is about pacing yourself, focusing on the task at hand, and avoiding too much tension and stress.

Your approach toward life is your philosophy. If you want a healthy lifestyle, a healthy philosophy toward fitness needs to be part of the picture. Remember that you already possess all that is required to successfully learn Yogilates—a changeable mind and body, an ability to learn, the power to create, and your own common sense. Ideally, your practice can be fun and invigorating, as well as serious and calming. Be open to a sense of wonder and enthusiasm as you discover hidden talents, and also be ready to tap into your own spirit for motivation and guidance.

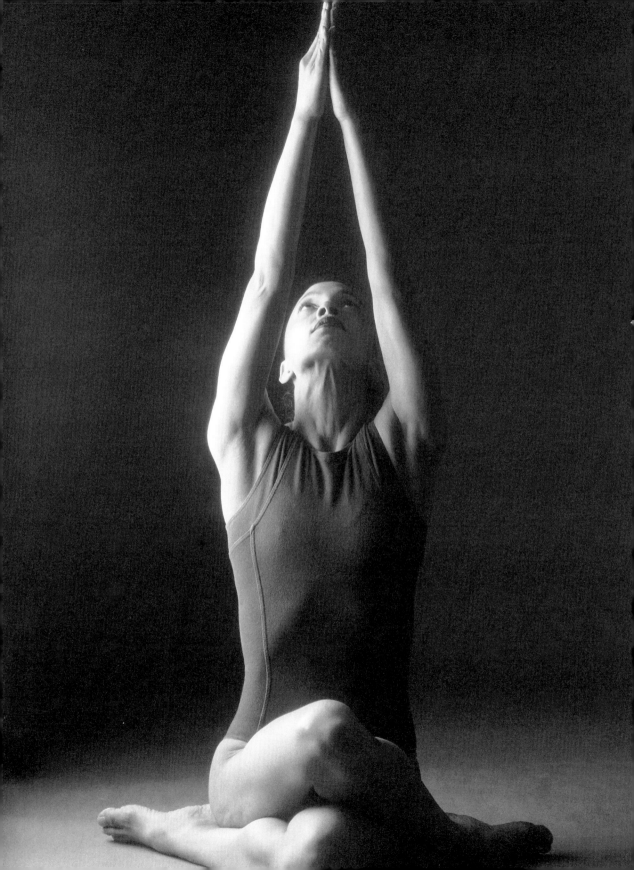

Chapter Two

From the Ground Up

Assessing Your Fitness Level

*"Your body is your first source of information
for developing proper fitness."*

We all have practical limits to what we can do with our bodies, and these things do not change overnight. Before beginning any exercise program, you should first understand what your present condition is and consider your previous exercise experience. Pushing yourself too far too soon is the most common cause of injury in exercise. Through a better understanding of the structure and mechanics of your body, you will be able to address your limitations with patience and common sense. Use this chapter to learn more about your body and to help you build a sound knowledge base from which to develop your practice.

Gravity is an equalizing force that has shaped the human body and governs its kinetics. From an evolutionary standpoint, our ability to rise up on our legs and free our hands for work is an example of overcoming

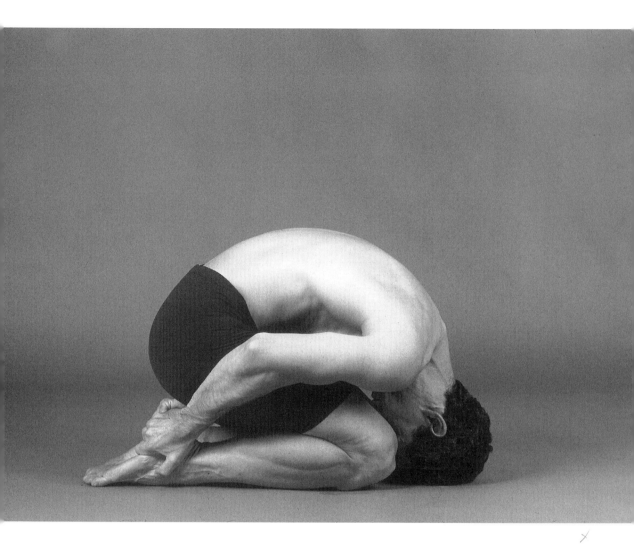

some of the limitations imposed by gravity. If you align your body efficiently, you can reduce the amount of energy you expend to fight against this constant force, and likewise minimize the wear and tear on your body. Basically, you have a choice when it comes to your relationship with gravity: you can support yourself consciously with good alignment, or you can support yourself unconsciously with gross posture. The latter is abusive to the body and can lead to big health problems down the road. Before assessing your posture, let's look at the three parts of your anatomy that have the greatest influence on skeletal alignment.

The Spine

Not all bodies are alike, but the human skeletal system is consistent in design and holds the key to your alignment. The central axis of your skeleton is the spine (Illustration 2.1). Think of your spine as a chain of joints that floats between two skeletal anchors, the pelvis and the skull, sort of like a Slinky toy. As you can see, the spine is slightly curved to help absorb shock and improve mobility. When you are standing or sitting, gravitational forces work to bring the two end points of your spine closer together, which, if not resisted through proper alignment and muscular support, can increase your spine's curvature and compress the spaces between the vertebrae. Through Yogilates, you will learn to articulate your spine and keep it flexible and strong.

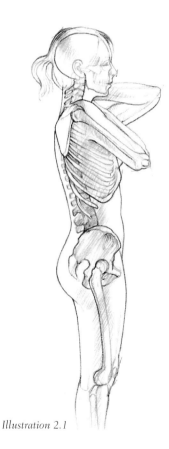

Illustration 2.1

The Pelvis

The pelvis is the largest bone in your body (Illustration 2.2) and has the largest and strongest muscles attached to it. Your ability to isolate and control your pelvis is key to the alignment of your torso and to stabilizing your spine. Think of your pelvis as the base on which the rest of your body's architecture is built. Your spine is connected to this base and supported by the surrounding musculature. Many chronic back problems originate from misalignment of the pelvis, which adversely affects the spine. Since Yogilates is a study of the body as well as a physical regimen, it helps to know the names and actions of the primary muscles involved with the pelvis, which include the abdominals, hip flexors and extensors, and lower back muscles. Your ability to engage these muscles to control the movement of your pelvis is key to establishing stability in your body. However, a more intuitive understanding of how to effectively use the core muscles around your pelvis will be gained simply by regularly performing the Yogilates exercises in this book.

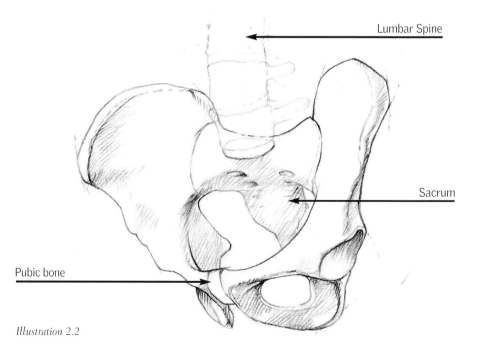

Lumbar Spine

Sacrum

Pubic bone

Illustration 2.2

The Shoulder Girdle

The shoulder girdle rests lightly on the top of the rib cage, with the clavicles stretching across the top of the chest and the scapula hanging from the back (Illustration 2.3). The shoulders can be moved independently or together and give tremendous mobility to the arms. Unfortunately, this floating quality to the shoulder girdle means that the shoulder joint can easily be destabilized during movements, thus increasing the risk of injury. In order to stabilize the shoulders, the muscles that connect the scapula to the ribs (middle trapezius and serratus) must be engaged. Also, the muscles on the front and back of the upper torso that connect the arms to the torso (primarily the latissimus and pectoralis muscles) must be strengthened, and the muscles that lift up on the shoulders from the neck (the trapezius and levators) deemphasized. Yogilates will teach you to control your range of motion and the quality of movement of your arms using your upper core muscles. This reduces unnecessary tension in the shoulders while adding control and stability to your upper body.

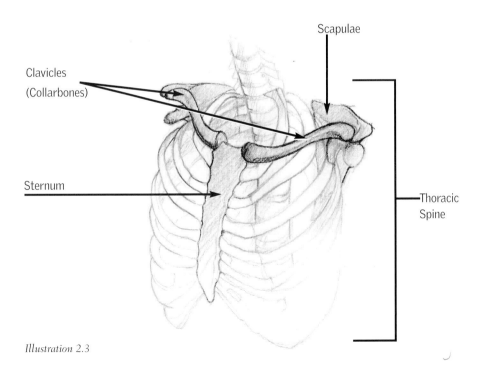

Illustration 2.3

Checking Your Posture

To check your posture, stand sideways in front of a mirror and look for the following landmarks: The ear in relation to the shoulder; the shoulder in relation to the side of the hip; the hip in relation to the knee; and the knee in relation to the ankle (photo 2.1). When you are in proper alignment, an imaginary plumb line connects the center points of all these landmarks. An extreme example of the breakdown of the body by gravity is a posture where the head is in front of the shoulders, the shoulders are behind the hips, the hips are tilted, and the knees are behind the ankles (photos 2.2 and 2.3). Look at yourself in the mirror to see if you have a tendency toward any of these imbalances.

Next, stand *facing* the mirror and notice the placement of your feet in relation to where your knees are. Look for any tilting to one side, either in the hips, shoulders, or head (photo 2.4). Common misalignments occur when the toes are pointed out rather than straight ahead, knees bow in, and one shoulder is higher than the other (photo 2.5).

Most of us carry some misalignment in our bodies either from bad habits, old injuries, or imbalanced muscular development. Fortunately, it is possible to correct most of these problems through symmetrical physical training—meaning working the whole body evenly. By helping you maintain focus on lengthening your spine, supporting with your core, and practicing precise alignment, Yogilates will give your body the structural integrity you need to achieve good posture for life. Within the first few weeks of your training, you will notice yourself standing and sitting taller, and moving with better balance and ease. Noting where you are *now* will make you appreciate the changes even more.

Test Your Flexibility

Lack of physical activity that moves through your range of motion, together with muscular tension associated with stress, gradually diminishes your flexibility over time. Tightness leads to a reduction in range of motion (ROM) which perpetuates more restrictions in other parts of the body. Fortunately, improving flexibility and ROM in all areas of the body is simply a matter of consistent effort and is built into the practice of Yogilates. But you need to get a sense of your present ROM to better understand your functional limits and to know when to utilize the appropriate modifications for some of the exercises. The following section will help you determine your starting flexibility in four key areas of your body: hamstrings, lower back, hip rotation, and shoulders. Test yourself in each area for current ROM and take note of clear restrictions.

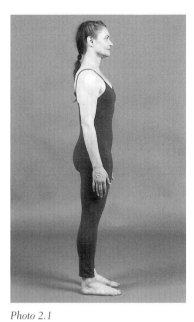

Photo 2.1

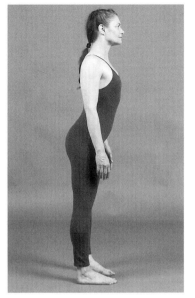

Photo 2.2

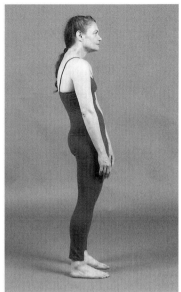

Photo 2.3

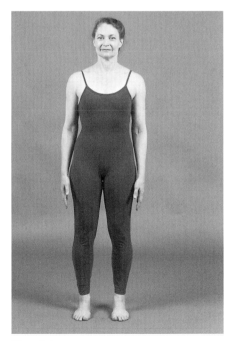

Photo 2.4

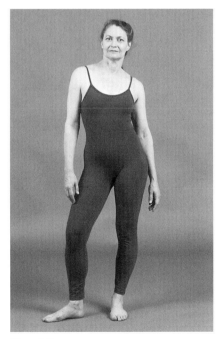

Photo 2.5

Hamstring Flexibility Test

Lie on your back with your arms by your sides. Lift one leg up to the ceiling without lifting your hip or bending the leg. Think of your leg moving along an arc of a compass, with a straight line to the ceiling being 90 degrees. Notice at what point you can no longer keep your leg straight. Also notice if the other leg wants to bend when you do this, or if it remains flat on the floor. If your leg goes up to 90 degrees, or beyond, quite easily without bending, then your hamstring on that leg is fairly loose.

Below are examples of restricted flexibility in the hamstring (photo 2.6) and unrestricted flexibility (photo 2.7).

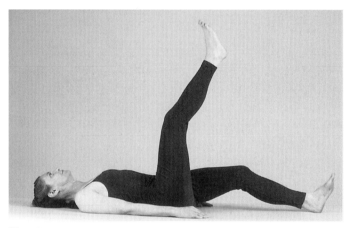

Photo 2.6

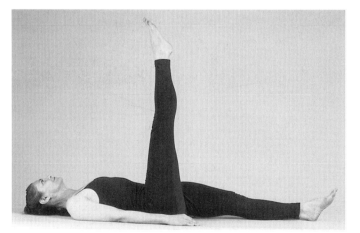

Photo 2.7

Suggested Exercises

While there are many ways to stretch the hamstring, this one is very safe because it doesn't put any strain on your lower back.

Lie on your back, bend your left leg and place the sole of your left foot flat on the floor. Using a rope 6 to 8 feet long or a yoga strap, make a loop around the bottom of your right foot and bend the knee into your chest. Hold the rope with both hands, supporting the weight of the leg with the rope. Then, leave your leg muscles as relaxed as possible as you exhale and use the rope to extend the right leg up toward the ceiling (photo 2.8). Inhale and bend it back down. Repeat stretching and bending your right leg ten times using the rope.

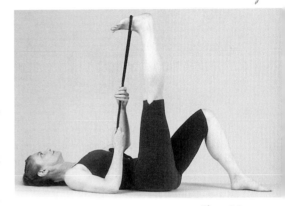

Photo 2.8

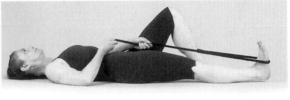

Photo 2.9

Next, keep your right leg as straight as you can without straining and, with the rope still looped around the foot, lower the leg a few inches from the floor (photo 2.9). Exhale and lift the right leg with the rope to whatever angle is possible without bending the knee or lifting the hips off the floor, feeling the stretch in your hamstring (photo 2.10). Supporting the leg with the rope, inhale and lower the right leg toward the floor again (photo 2.11). Repeat lowering and raising the right leg with the breath 10 times.

Change the rope to the left leg and repeat both assisted leg stretches.

If you do these exercises once a day for several weeks, you should notice a gradual improvement in your hamstring flexibility. Eventually, you should be able to do these exercises with the non-working leg flat on the floor instead of bent.

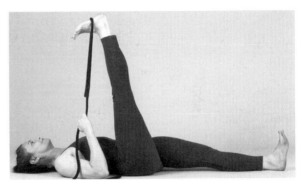

Photo 2.10

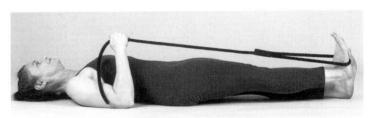

Photo 2.11

Lower-Back Flexibility Test

Stand about a foot and a half from a wall, bend your knees a little, and sit back against the wall with your arms by your sides (photo 2.12). Starting from the top of your head, exhale and slowly roll down, trying to peel your back off the wall one vertebra at a time. Pause after you have rolled halfway down, with just your shoulders and upper back off the wall (photo 2.13). Notice if you can keep the middle and lower back on the wall while your upper torso is in a full curve forward. If this is difficult, it indicates tightness in the upper parts of your spine.

Inhale during the pause, then exhale and continue rolling down, allowing your torso to fully bend over your legs (you may support yourself with your hands on your thighs). Keep your buttocks leaning against the wall and notice how close your chest and stomach can get to your thighs. The photo on the left illustrates restricted flexion in the lower back (photo 2.14), while the right shows unrestricted flexion (photo 2.15). To come out of this position, place your hands on your thighs and exhale as you roll back up to standing.

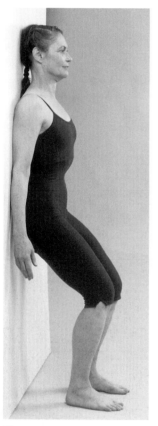

Photo 2.12

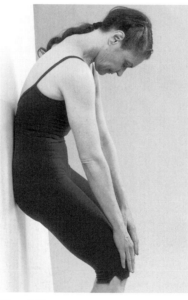

Photo 2.13

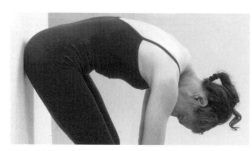

Photo 2.14

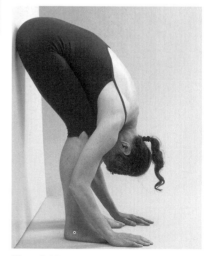

Photo 2.15

Suggested Exercise

Practice the standing roll-down (Page 26) against the wall 3 times, pausing for 3 breaths in the halfway position, and proceeding to the full bent-over position (photos 2.16 and 2.17). Breathe deeply for 3 to 5 breaths in the last position to help stretch out your spine. Move slowly and give your body weight over to gravity, allowing your head to let go and your back muscles to lengthen.

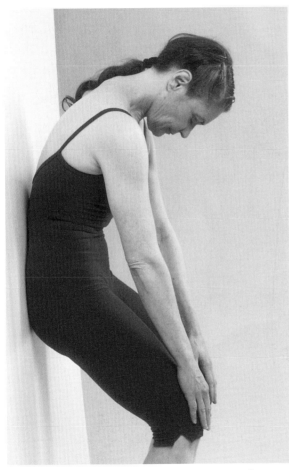

Photo 2.16

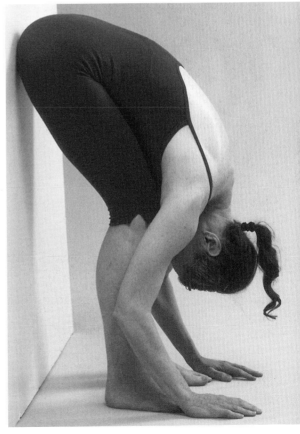

Photo 2.17

Hip Rotation Flexibility Test

Sit on the floor and bend your legs in, placing the soles of your feet together. If it is difficult to sit with a straight back you may sit up on a firm pillow or folded blanket. Place your hands on the floor and allow your legs to relax and your knees to fall open. Notice how high your knees are from the ground (photos 2.18 and 2.19). On the left is an example of restriction in the hip rotators; the right indicates unrestricted mobility.

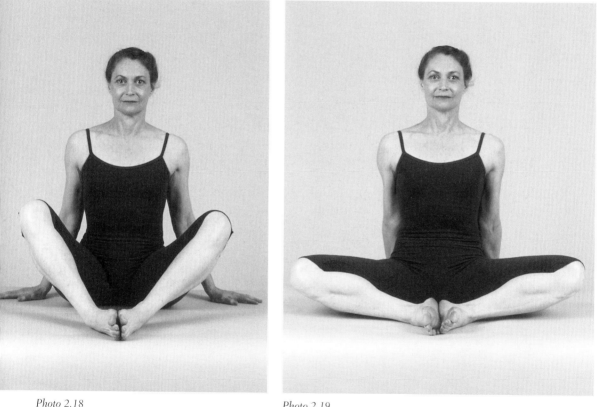

Photo 2.18

Photo 2.19

Suggested Exercise

Lie on your back and scoot your seat up next to a wall. Place the legs up on the wall and bring the soles of the feet together as when you were sitting for the test (photo 2.20). Place your hands on the inside of your knees and exhale as you gently press the thighs open. Then, inhale and press the thighs in against your hands for resistance. Repeat this sequence 5 times using long, full breaths, letting the leg and hip muscles release a little more open every time you exhale.

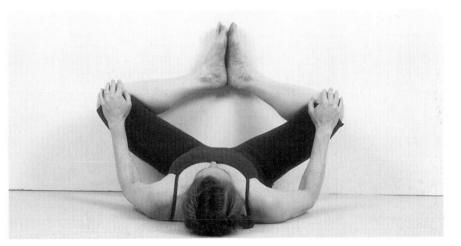

Photo 2.20

Shoulder Flexibility Test

Stand with your back flat up against a wall and place your right arm in a 90-degree bend out from your shoulder, fingers pointing to the ceiling (photo 2.21). Try to keep your arm flat against the wall while also keeping your back and shoulder blades flat.

Exhale as you slowly slide the arm up along the wall toward the ceiling, again trying to maintain the back and shoulders flat on the wall (photos 2.22 and 2.23). The photo on the left demonstrates restriction in the shoulders, where the right is unrestricted.

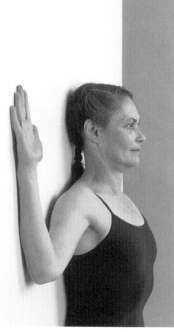

Photo 2.21

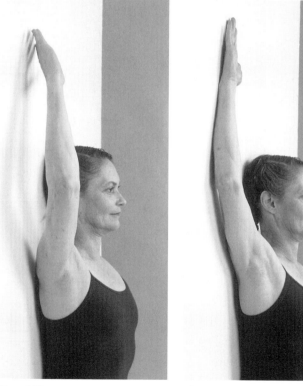

Photo 2.22   *Photo 2.23*

Suggested Exercise

Using a rope or yoga strap, stand and hold it with your hands slightly wider than your shoulders. Inhale and raise your arms straight over your head. Then, exhale and slowly reach your arms behind you and down without bending your arms. Adjust your grip wider if necessary to where you can circle your arms all the way down behind you and back up without needing to bend your arms (photos 2.24 and 2.25). Inhale and bring your arms back over your head. Repeat this assisted arm circle 10 times, feeling a good stretch in the shoulders and chest area. You will notice that it gets easier after the first few times.

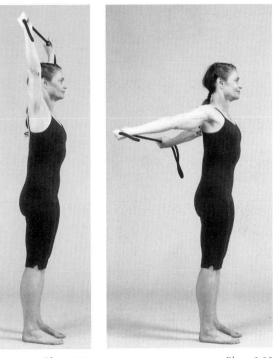

Photo 2.24   *Photo 2.25*

It is important to remember that, as with postural imbalances, all the range-of-motion restrictions depicted in the preceding pages are common for most people. Most of us will have some restriction in these areas, and you should not be critical of yourself if you do. This is just your starting point. Focusing on what you can't do will only impede your progress, and you may end up fighting against yourself. Sometimes, the effort necessary to improve posture or range of motion is about using less force and relaxing all over, rather than trying harder. Yogilates is about expanding your physical potential and awareness, not about achieving perfect flexibility. Overreaching in a stretch, or holding a pose too long, are two of the most common ways people get injured in yoga and Pilates. The wise student knows that staying within the boundaries of his or her abilities will actually allow them to advance rapidly *and* safely at the same time.

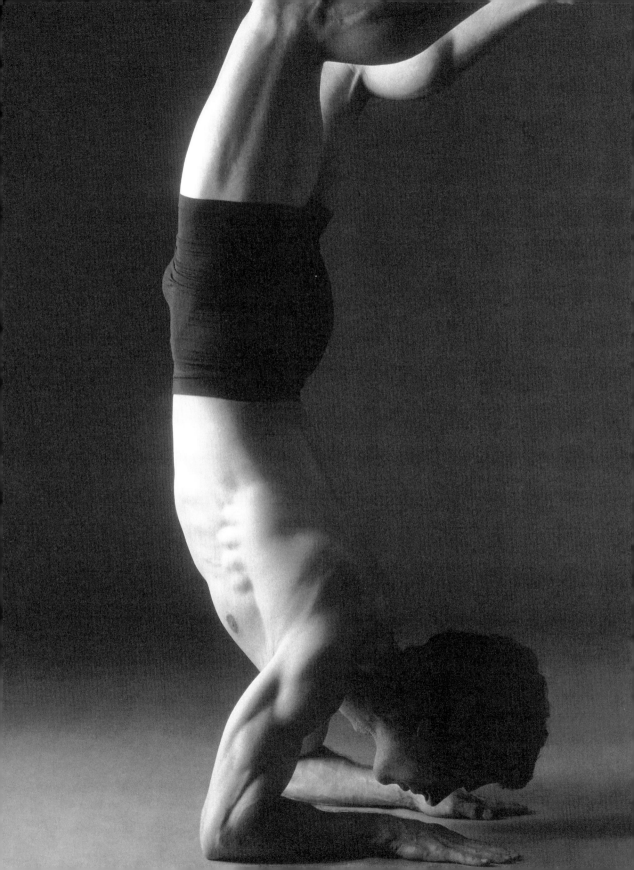

Chapter Three

The Yogilates Essential Awareness Exercises

Sound exercise technique and consistent practice go hand in hand and provide the living structure behind Yogilates. In this chapter, you will learn the fundamental principles of Yogilates technique and how to apply them to functional movements with your body. You will also be introduced to a vocabulary of useful images and sensory cues that will help guide your intuitive understanding of the technique as you refine your skills.

First, we will look at the science of breathing efficiently, which includes isolating the diaphragm and controlling the depth of your breath cycle. Next, we will discover where your core muscles are and how they are used in Yogilates technique. In the second section, you will learn the 10 Essential Awareness Exercises of Yogilates. These exercises encapsulate the central principles of Yogilates technique, teaching you breath technique, how to establish proper alignment, how to effectively engage the core muscles and how to control movement from your center. Do not skip this portion of the book; these exercises are vital to understanding, progressing, and exercising safely in your Yogilates practice.

Breathing, the Diaphragm, and the Core

More than your need for oxygen, how you breathe at any given moment is related to your instinctual responses to your environment and to your changing emotional states. Most of your breathing is done unconsciously, which is why breathing incorrectly is such a difficult habit to break. When most people are asked to breathe they naturally think of inhaling. But breathing is clearly a two-part operation: the inhalation and the exhalation. Emphasis on inhalation leads to "overbreathing," which can cause tension, hyperventilation and lightheadedness. The truth is we all carry around more air than we actually need and people frequently overinflate their chests and abdominal areas with excess air. This creates myriad imbalances, including tight muscles in the chest and back, distension of the belly, and misalignment. During exercise, the internal pressure from being partially blown up can give you an artificial sense of support in the torso. Relying on this is dangerous because as soon as the air is expelled, that support vanishes. Over-breathing also pushes the rib cage out to the front, taking the spine with it.

In Yogilates, you will focus on the full breath cycle, completing full exhalations so that your chest and back relax, and your spine can maintain proper alignment. Notice the next time you let out a good sigh how this deep exhalation helps release tension and lengthen your body out.

Joseph Pilates believed that emphasizing exhalation when breathing helped to expunge the impure air that resides in the bottom of your lungs. He was right. Only when you completely exhale can air in the lower lobes of the lungs get pushed out, thus allowing clean fresh air to be brought in.

In yoga, the aim is to ensure that an even tide of air flows in and out of the lungs. The hatha yoga practices of Ujjayi breathing, which involves restricting the flow of air by slightly closing the back of the throat, and Pranayama, which involves breathing strongly and deeply through one nostril and holding the breath, develop stronger breathing muscles and maintain internal focus. Apart from helping rid the body of toxins and exercising the breathing muscles, consciously working on your breath helps center the mind and relieve stress.

A yogi would say your breath is the thread that ties all your asanas together and unites your being with the higher spirit. Listening to my breath while doing Yogilates reminds me of the philosophy behind my practice: appreciate it (without it I can't live), be present (it goes on all the time), be moderate (if my breathing is labored, I'm working too hard), and enjoy it (breathing well is living well).

The Diaphragm

The most natural and most efficient way to breathe is with your diaphragm, which is located just below the bottom of your lungs inside the lower ribs (Illustration 3.1). You can't see or touch your diaphragm, but you can feel it pull down to bring in air and release up to push air out of the lungs. Contrary to what you might think, the ribs are not fixed, but are attached with hinge joints to the spine so that they can expand to accommodate full breathing, much like an umbrella opening and closing (Illustration 3.2).

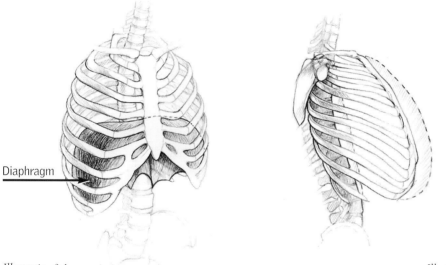

Diaphragm

Illustration 3.1   *Illustration 3.2*

The Core Muscles

Exercises that simply target the abdominals are not what the core is all about. The core muscles you should concentrate on are deeper than the surface abdominals and wrap around the lower torso and hips like a wide cummerbund. Core muscles also include the smaller internal muscles that connect the inside of the ribs, and hold the shoulder blades in place. In Yogilates, you will learn to stabilize your body (particularly your pelvis, spine, ribs, and shoulder girdle) as well as direct all your movements from these centrally located muscles. Surface muscles are to be relaxed so that you connect to the inner roots of your body, allowing your spine, your legs, and your arms to float as extensions from your center. By focusing your effort from within, the strength and power are hidden, hence the Pilates phrase "hidden powerhouse." The face, neck, hands and feet are to be relaxed so that extraneous tension is dissipated and an appearance of grace and effortlessness is created.

The Essential Awareness Exercises

To help you master the fundamental principles of Yogilates technique, I created the following Essential Awareness Exercises. With regular practice, these exercises help you breathe efficiently, maintain proper alignment, release unnecessary tension, and integrate your core muscles into your movement. These skills are essential to understanding Yogilates technique and will be referred to again and again throughout the book.

Each exercise is described in terms of its lesson, which regards the skill you will be working on, and is then broken down in terms of physical and mental preparation and action. At the end, there is additional instruction, called "refinement," to provide a deeper understanding of the technique using visual and sensory imagery.

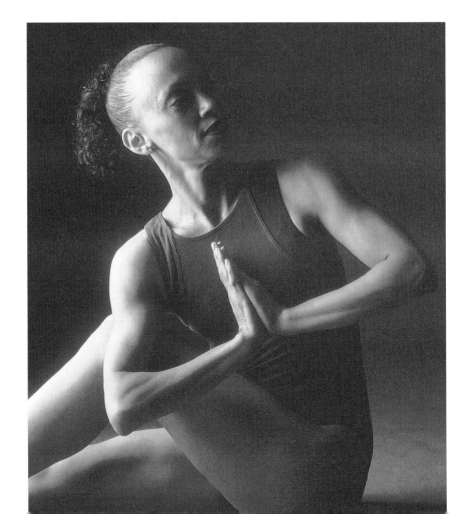

1. Symmetrical Rib-Cage Breathing

Lesson: How to place the breath in the diaphragm and the ribs

Preparation: Sit on a firm pillow with the legs crossed and your back supported by a wall or couch. Place your hands on the sides of your ribs (photo 3.1). Sitting tall, keep your mouth closed and breath just through your nose.

Action: Take 2 full breaths, feeling your ribs expand out to the sides as you inhale and contract in as you exhale. Relax your chest and resist letting the belly expand out with the intake. This creates symmetrical rib-cage breathing on either side of the body and avoids any distorting effect on the spine.

Refinement: On your next breath, extend the exhalation for 3 to 5 counts and use your hands to gently help push out all your air. Feel your abdominals pressing in, and don't be afraid to completely lose your breath. On the subsequent inhale you should feel your diaphragm pulling the air in from deep in your torso. Practice these full exhalations for 3 more breath cycles, being careful to expand the ribs only to the sides and not to the front.

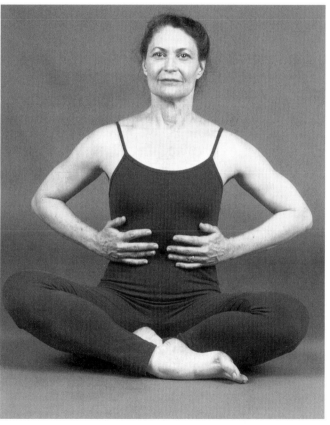

Photo 3.1

2. Pilates Lip Breathing

Lesson: How to exhale with resistance through the lips

Preparation: Sit as you did in the previous exercise and rest your hands on your thighs (photo 3.2). Keep breathing with the diaphragm and the ribs.

Action 1: Inhale through the nose and then exhale completely through slightly parted lips, blowing the air down the front of your body (photo 3.3). Your mouth should be shaped just as if you were blowing on the top of a bottle to make it whistle. Feel how the resistance of expelling air through your lips makes your torso muscles work. Be mindful not to puff your cheeks or make a hissing sound as you do this. Practice this Pilates lip breathing for 4 breath cycles.

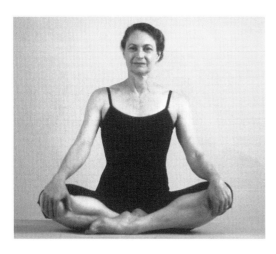

Photo 3.2

3. Ujjayi Breathing

Lesson: Full cycle breathing against resistance

Preparation: Same as above

Action 1: Breathing just through your nose, partially close the back of your throat to make a slight snoring sound as you breath. This is called Ujjayi breathing, and you should feel resistance to the passage of air during both the inhalation and exhalation. Practice for 4 complete breath cycles.

Refinement: Practice both styles of resistance breathing for one minute trying to extend the length of your breaths from 6 to 10 counts. Do this with your eyes closed to heighten your awareness of the placement and effort of your breathing. After you stop, breathe easily through the nose for one minute, keeping your back straight and feeling your ribs gently opening and closing with your breath.

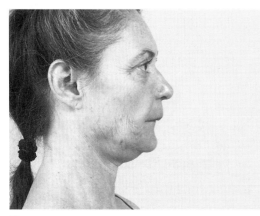

Photo 3.3

(**Note:** For all remaining Essential Awareness Exercises, breathe through the nose in an even pace, coordinated with the actions as instructed.)

4. Pelvic Tilts and Imprinting

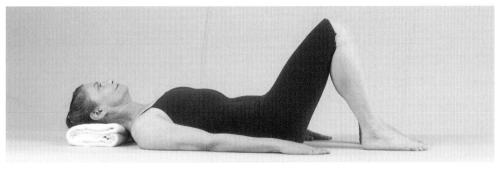

Photo 3.4

Lesson: How to isolate your pelvis and stabilize your spine

Preparation: Lie on your back with your legs bent so both feet are flat on the floor, hip-width apart, and place your arms by your sides. If necessary, place a folded towel under your head to help keep your head from tilting back (photo 3.4). With your hand, locate your pubic bone at the lower front of your pelvis, and your two hipbones to the sides of your lower stomach. Also, take note of the slight curve of your lower back off the ground.

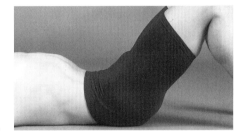

Photo 3.5

Action 1: Tilt your pubic bone up just enough to flatten the curve in your lower back. Don't push your hips up or tuck so much that your tailbone curls off the floor. Then tilt the pubic bone down, exaggerating the arch of your lower back off the floor (photos 3.5 and 3.6). Repeat, tilting your pelvis each way 6 times, exhaling out of the belly as you tilt the pubic bone up and inhaling into the belly as you tilt it down.

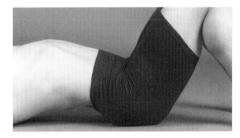

Photo 3.6

Action 2: Tilt the pubic bone up again and stay there. Exhale completely and relax the lower stomach, allowing it to fully deflate and sink down to the back (photo 3.7). Keep your belly hollowed out and breathe just to the sides of your ribs. With your back flat and the belly deflated, this is referred to as "imprinting" the back. Practice 4 breath cycles in this position.

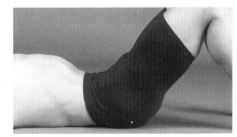

Photo 3.7

5. Hip Twists and Neutral Pelvis

Lesson: How to establish the pelvis in a neutral position

Preparation: From the pelvis tilt above, release the tilt and allow the pelvis to return to a neutral position between the two tilts. Place your hands on your hips during this exercise for greater awareness.

Action 1: Tilt the left side of your pelvis up and the right side down without engaging your leg muscles (photo 3.8). If you were standing, this would be like twisting your hips to the right. Return to level and then tilt the right side up. Repeat, alternating side tilts with the pelvis 3 times each side and then return to level.

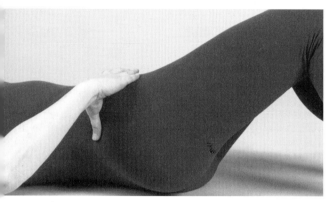

Photo 3.8

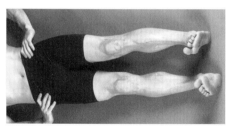

Photo 3.9

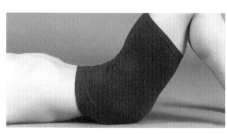

Photo 3.10

Action 2: Extend both legs out on the floor while keeping the pelvis from tilting forward or back or to any one side. Then, reach down farther with the right leg and hip, pulling the left side of your hip up toward your left rib (photo 3.9). This creates a diagonal tilt in the hips, and you should feel the muscles on the lower right side of your back elongate and the muscles on the lower left side of your back contract. These are your quadratus muscles, also know as your "hip hikers" because they lift up your hips from the sides. Bring the right leg and hip back to level with the left, and then repeat the diagonal tilt the other way. Reach down with your left hip and up with the right.

Refinement: Bend in your legs and place the feet flat on the floor. Take a moment to sense the control you have to tilt your pelvis forward and back and side to side, and to reach it away or up from the sides. Ideally, the pelvis should feel like it is hanging down in a neutral position, level at all angles and free from any tilting (photo 3.10). Visualize the space between your lower ribs and the sides of your hips, and feel how this helps your lower spine feel longer.

6. Knee Folds

Lesson: How to lift the legs in to you using the core muscles

Preparation: Lie on your back with your legs bent so that both feet are flat on the floor, and place your arms by your sides. If necessary, place a folded towel under your head to help keep your head from arching back (photo 3.11).

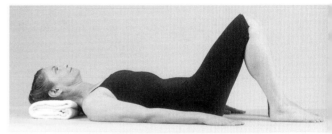

Photo 3.11

Action 1: Draw your navel to your spine and exhale as you lift one knee toward your chest. Leave the leg fully bent and completely relaxed so you bring it into you with your core muscles and not the thigh. Working softly with the leg, it should feel like it "folds" into the crease of the front of your hip. Inhale and set it back down. Repeat with the other leg. Watch that the leg stays in parallel alignment and the pelvis stays neutral. Alternate knee folds 10 times (photos 3.12 and 3.13).

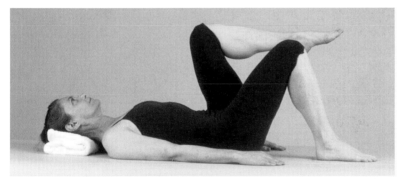

Photo 3.12

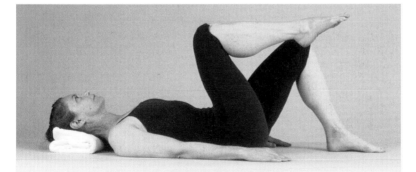

Photo 3.13

7. Toe Touches

Lesson: How to move the legs away from you using the core muscles

Preparation: Fold both knees in to your chest, leaving your legs completely bent and relaxed. Point your toes and place your hands under the bottom edge of your hips (photos 3.14 and 3.15).

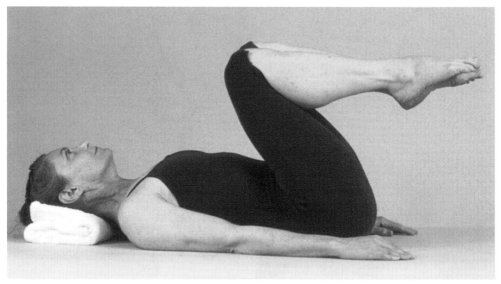

Photo 3.14

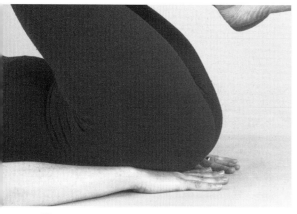

Photo 3.15

Action 1: Feeling your back "imprinted," exhale as you lower one foot to touch the floor with your toes. Control the action with your core muscles deep in your lower abdominal area. Inhale and bring the foot back up. Repeat with the other leg (photo 3.16). Alternate toe touches slowly 10 times, keeping your thighs parallel and close to each other as your move them.

Action 2: Keeping your legs fully bent and the back imprinted, exhale strongly to help compress the lower abdominals and slowly lower both feet to just touch the floor with your toes. Inhale and bring them back up (photo 3.17). Repeat double toe touches 5 times.

This is much harder than single toe touches, as you now have to control the weight of both legs from your core while maintaining the back imprinted and the belly hollowed.

Refinement: Notice that as the legs move away from your center, the lower back will want to release from the floor and the abdominals may push up. Don't let them! Try to tilt your pubic bone up in opposition to the legs moving away in order to keep the back flat and the stomach down.

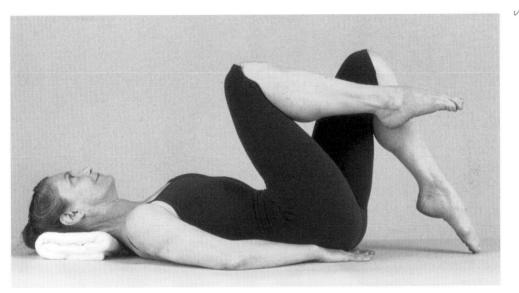

Photo 3.16

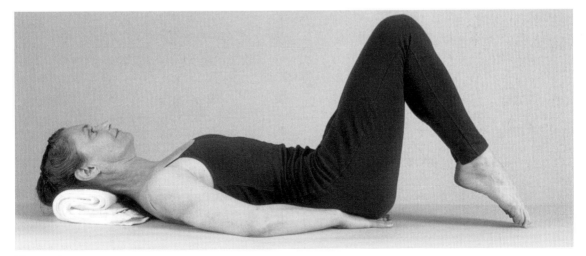

Photo 3.17

8. Arm Reaches

Lesson: To improve awareness of the shoulder girdle and shoulder blades

Preparation: Lie on your back with the legs bent, feet flat on the floor and hip-width apart. Reach both arms straight to the ceiling with the palms facing each other. Start with both shoulder blades down and flat on the floor.

Action: Inhale and reach one arm and shoulder up off the ground. Exhale and lower the shoulder back down (photos 3.18 and 3.19). Alternate single-arm reaches 5 times. Then, inhale and reach up with both arms and shoulders, and exhale as you lower. Repeat double-arm reaches 5 times. Feel your shoulder blades flatten onto the ground each time you lower from a reach.

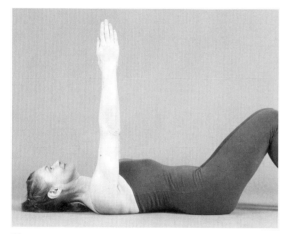

Photo 3.18

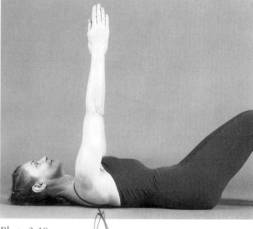

Photo 3.19

9. Arm Circles

Lesson: How to move the arms through a range of motion without destabilizing the shoulder joint

Preparation: Lie on your back with the legs bent, feet flat on the floor, and place both arms by your sides, palms down. Keep your arms straight and palms and fingers stretched long throughout this exercise.

Action: Inhale and slowly lift the arms out along the ground to shoulder height (Illustration 3.3). Then rotate the palms up, and continue lifting the arms over your head as you exhale. Don't let the weight of the arms pull your middle back off the ground or hike your shoulders up.

Next, inhale and lift your arms from overhead to the ceiling with the palms facing in. Exhale as you lower them back down to your side. Repeat the arm circle in the same direction, and then reverse the direction of the circle 2 times.

Refinement: Engage the muscles under your arms, and around your rib cage, in opposition to the movement of the arms away from your center. Your goal is to let the arms feel long and relaxed as you move them smoothly around with muscles inside the chest and back. Feel your shoulder blades like two flat plates connected to the floor, unaffected by the arm circles.

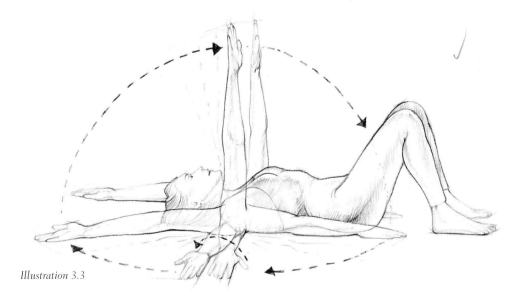

Illustration 3.3

10. Neutral Stance and Small Knee Bends

Lesson: How to engage the core muscles while standing in proper alignment. (You will need a 12-inch ruler.)

Preparation: Stand with your feet hip-width apart and in parallel position, meaning your

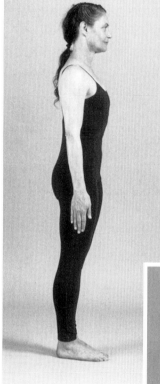

Photo 3.20

toes are pointing forward (photo 3.20). To make sure your feet are the right distance apart, locate the two bones on the front of your hips. Using a ruler, hold it on one end and let it hang down vertically. Place the side of the ruler on your right hipbone and look down the line of the ruler to the floor (photo 3.21). Align the middle toe of your right foot with that line. Do the same on the left side. For most people, this means the distance between your feet will be around 5 to 8 inches apart, with women having a generally wider stance than men. This is your "neutral stance." Set the ruler down, place your hands on your hips and feel yourself centered over your feet.

Action: Inhale as you do a small knee bend, keeping the knees in line with the feet (photo 3.22). Be aware not to take your pelvis forward with your knees (photo 3.23). Exhale to straighten back up, being careful not to lock the knees straight (photo 3.24). Repeat the small knee bends 8 times.

Refinement: Allow your buttocks, lower back, and hip muscles to relax and bring the lower abdominals in. When you're standing, your pelvis should feel like it is hanging straight down with the tailbone dropping like a plumb line to the ground. Feel your feet connected to the floor, releasing your weight down into the ground. Then imagine that you have another pair of feet under your hips that are just as connected to the ground. As you do the small knee bends, imag-

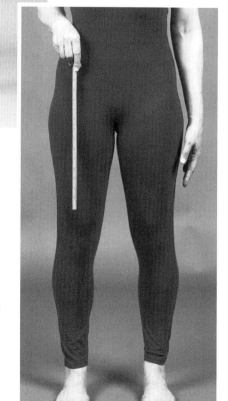

Photo 3.21

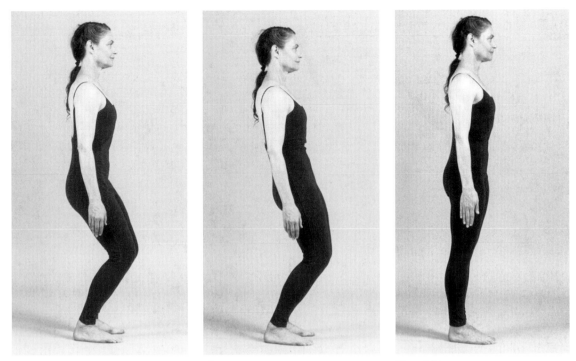

Photo 3.22   Photo 3.23   Photo 3.24

ine initiating the action from these "hip-high feet." Feel how this image engages your core muscles while your thigh muscles and knees become less involved. Being able to feel grounded and bending and straightening your legs with assistance from your core muscles will reduce stress on your joints and will help you move with more grace and power from your center during all your standing exercises.

———————

By reading and doing the exercises in this chapter consistently, you will gain the knowledge and awareness necessary for proceeding in your Yogilates practice. The sensations you experience and the imagery you create while exploring these fundamental exercises will become a part of your personal Yogilates wisdom. Try to use some of the skills and visualizations you learned in the Essential Awareness Exercises in your everyday living. Focus on your breathing to help reduce feelings of tension or stress. Notice the alignment of your pelvis when you are standing and sitting. Feel the strength in your core help you to get up from the couch or into the car. Explore your range of motion with your arms when you reach around yourself as you bathe. Translating the awareness you gain from Yogilates to everyday consciousness will help you find meaningful purpose and devotion to your practice.

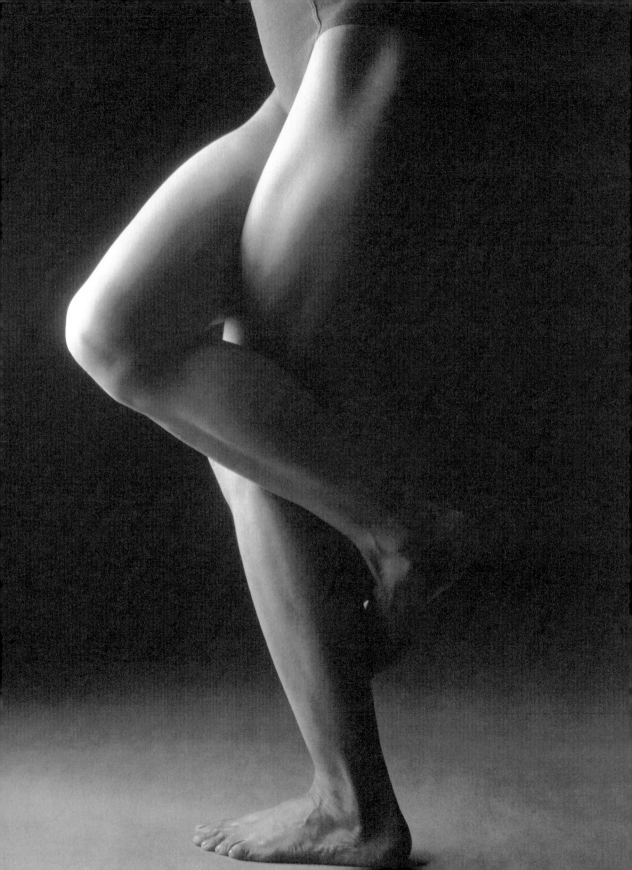

Chapter Four

The Beginner Series

The physical act of repeated practice can be
considered an excellent sacred mentor.

—Jerry Lynch and Chungliang Huang,
Working Out, Working Within

Y ou are now ready to learn a complete Yogilates routine that will provide you a daily regimen to start your practice. Remember to never push or strain to achieve any position, or an injury may result. Be patient with yourself and study the accompanying photographs for each exercise before you do it. Read all the instructions and take note of the modifications as well. Yogilates creates change in your body over time. Consistent practice with particular awareness to the breath and to the correct alignment of your body is what you should focus on rather than the intensity of muscular effort. Then one day, while you are enjoying the experience of your practice, you will notice that a difficult pose is suddenly easier, and you have gone a bit farther or deeper. In Yogilates practice, allow the changes to come to you like a gift you wanted but were not really expecting.

Frequently Asked Questions About Yogilates

How often should I practice Yogilates?

Yogilates exercises are nourishing to the body, calming to the mind, and can be done every day. I recommend performing the Beginner Series at least 3 times a week to start. As you become more experienced, you may practice a full routine 5 times a week. Remember to regularly give your body a rest to allow for complete recovery and for the changes in your neurological pathways to be absorbed. Never giving your body a break can actually retard your progress and significantly increase the risk of injury.

How long does the routine take?

Although referring to the instructions at first will make things go slower, once you become familiar with the exercises, the Beginner Series should normally take you 30 to 40 minutes to complete.

How do I know if I'm doing Yogilates correctly?

As I mentioned before, a mirror is a valuable tool for checking the alignment of your positions. If you have a partner to practice with, you can take turns helping each other with your form. If you diligently practice your Essential Awareness Exercises, most of the information you need to assess your form and technique will come from how the exercises feel.

For example, pay attention to the quality of your breathing. If your breathing becomes shallow or halting it is a sign to ease up. Likewise, if your muscles start to cramp or quiver, or your shoulders or hips become tense, these are signs that your technique is off and you should pause and correct yourself. The goal is to move through the exercises with a sense of ease, balance, and control. You should also select and modify the exercises as appropriate for your level. Even if you could do only half the series at first, as long as you brought your full attention to it and you breathed, then it was magic and your practice was a success.

Is it okay to do more repetitions or hold the positions for longer than directed?

Do no more or no fewer reps than specified, and there is no need to hold positions longer than recommended. Naturally, your tendency will be to do more reps or spend more time on those exercises that you find easy and less on those that are difficult. This tendency will only add to your imbalance. Remember that Yogilates is about quality and moderation, performing just enough to create an elegant balance in the body in terms of muscular development and coordination.

How do I know when I'm ready to progress to the next level of Yogilates?

Like any skill that is worth learning, Yogilates must be practiced over and over to master. Repetition of the basics does more to create lasting changes in your mind and your body than performing a difficult pose once in a while. Remember that you are not only practicing the exercises but also practicing your awareness skills. Once your routine is fully memorized, and may even feel monotonous, immerse yourself in the process of the moment and just feel what is happening in your body. Take time to focus on connecting to your breath and to receive more feedback from your body about your strengths and weaknesses. That increase in your awareness is the first way you progress in Yogilates. Then, when you are performing the full routine smoothly with complete control and ease, you can consider progressing to the more advanced exercises.

Do I need any special clothing or equipment?

You need enough floor space to do the exercises, a yoga mat to protect your back and keep your hands and feet from slipping, a rolled towel to place under your head, and a firm pillow to sit on. In addition, a yoga strap, 2- or 3-pound dumbbells, and a

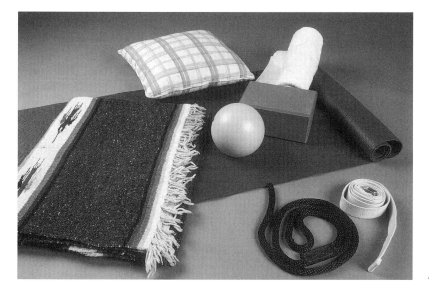

Photo 4.1

foam yoga block can be used for some exercises (photo 4.1). Wear loose clothing, such as a T-shirt and shorts, or a unitard. Remove shoes, socks, and dangling jewelry. You need to be barefoot to work the feet effectively and to secure footing on the mat.

What else might enhance my Yogilates practice?

Choose a time when it is quiet and you can concentrate. Digestive activity can affect your breathing and circulation, so it is best not to eat for at least two hours prior to practice.

Practice under soft lighting, although any lighting will work as long as you avoid direct light in your eyes. Some people enjoy candlelight for evening practice.

Keep the room comfortably warm (72°–76°F). In a slightly warm environment, your body will be more pliable and your muscles more relaxed. But again, don't think more is better. Higher temperatures are not necessary or more beneficial and can strain your system.

At first, practice Yogilates in silence, which will heighten your awareness of your breathing. Once you have memorized your routine, you may like to have music on to help provide rhythm and inspiration to your practice. Instrumental music appropriate for practice should be carefully selected so as not to be distracting. Silence or ambient music played very softly is recommended for meditation.

It is an inherent weakness of any exercise book that the photos are of static positions, showing a beginning and an end. The routine has been choreographed so that each exercise leads to the next. Visualize bringing the pictures to life and see yourself gracefully connecting the positions to one another.

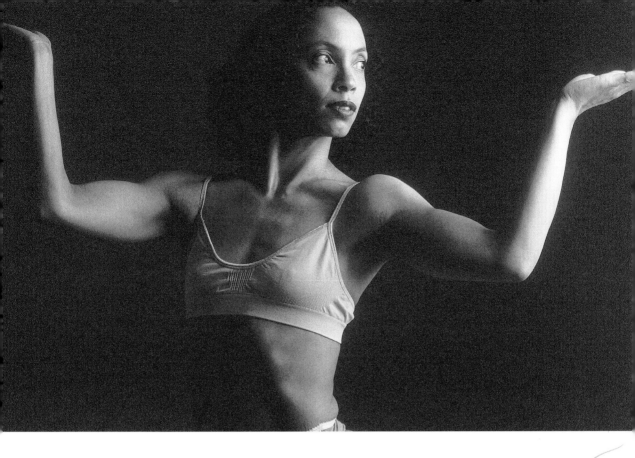

Breathing Techniques

The appropriate breathing style for each exercise is given at the beginning of each exercise. Breathing fully with the diaphragm through the nose is the normal instruction for most exercises. However, when a more complete exhalation to help compress the abdominal area is desired, the recommended style is in the Pilates manner. When more intense breathing with resistance is desired, Ujjayi breathing is directed.

Except for a few specifically noted instances, your breathing should always be placed in the sides of your ribs with the belly hollowed out, navel to spine. Connect to your breath first and then let the action happen. You should always feel a suspension-expansion during the inhalation and a release-deepening of the stretch during the exhalation.

Special note: Look for the symbol ☯, which will denote modifications for exercises or positions you may find difficult.

1. Easy Pose Warm-Up

Ujjayi breathing through the nose

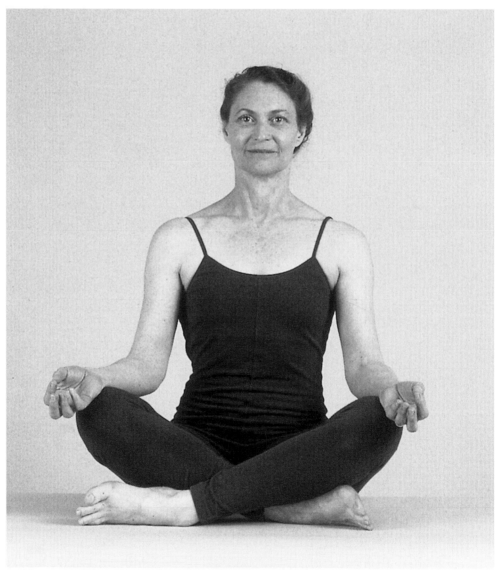

Photo 4.2

☯ *If sitting up straight in this pose is difficult, try extending the legs out halfway and using a firm pillow to raise your seat a few inches off the ground (photo 4.3).*

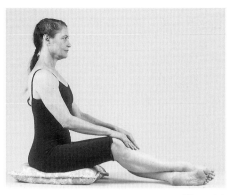

Sitting on your mat with your legs crossed, lightly hold on to your shins and lift your spine up as tall and as long as you can (photo 4.4). Visualize the entire length of your spine unfurling from your tailbone to the top of your head.

Let go of your shins and place the backs of your hands on your knees. Close your eyes and circle your shoulders backward 4 times; breath in as you circle up and out as you circle down. On the last circle, exhale fully and let your shoulders relax down. Soften your chest and feel your ribs fall down and in.

Photo 4.3

Place the breath in the sides of your ribs with the lower abdominals pulled in, and do slow Ujjayi breathing for 5 breath cycles (photo 4.5). Center your mind's eye on following your breath as you allow distracting thoughts or worries to fade away.

Visualize a point on your spine equal in height to where your navel is. Inhale to that spot and feel your back lengthen up and down from this spot. This will naturally draw the navel to the spine without tensing or contracting the surface abdominals. When you exhale, just feel the front and back of the body coming closer together.

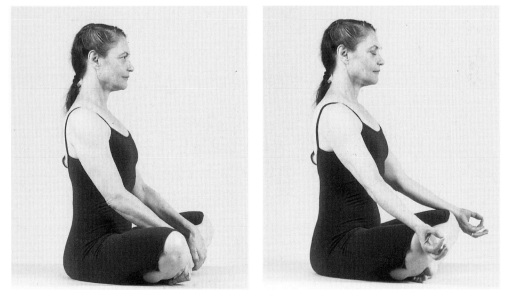

Photo 4.4

Photo 4.5

2. Arm Breaths and Side Curves

normal diaphragmatic breathing through the nose

Open your eyes and reach your arms down straight (photo 4.6). Focus on your breathing as you lift your arms overhead with the inhalation (photo 4.7), and press them down as you exhale. Keep your back straight, the ribs in place, and the shoulders down. Repeat Arm Breaths 3 times.

Next, reach up one arm with your inhale, and then curve to the side as you exhale, catching yourself with the hand and forearm of your other arm (photos 4.8 and 4.9). Alternate sides, curving over twice to each side.

❷ *If reaching the arm up and over creates tension in your shoulders or neck, leave the arms by your sides, and just curve with the torso.*

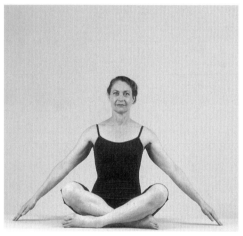

Photo 4.6

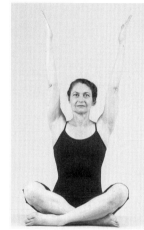

Photo 4.7

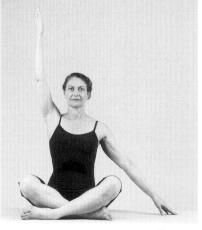

Photo 4.8

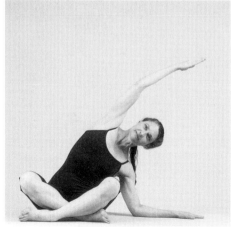

Photo 4.9

3. Back Scoops

exhaling through the lips in the Pilates manner

Sit with the soles of the feet together, knees out to the sides. Place your hands on your shins (photo 4.10). Exhale as you round your spine, scoop in your abdomen, and engage your buttocks. Inhale to bring your back up straight (photo 4.11). Repeat Back Scoops 3 times.

When I work with this exercise, I imagine that my back is a sail and the wind comes along and catches it, rounding my torso back and spreading it full and wide. Allow your head to relax forward and be sure not to hunch your shoulders.

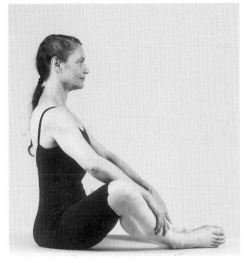

Photo 4.10

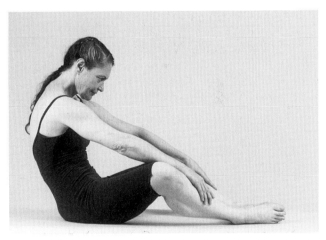

Photo 4.11

4. Sternum Lifts

normal diaphragmatic breathing through the nose

Place your hands right behind your hips, fingers pointing to the back. Inhale as you push down strongly with your arms and arch your sternum up to the ceiling (photo 4.12). Be careful not to hyperextend your elbows. Exhale to return to sitting straight. Repeat Sternum Lift again.

To maximize the stretch in the chest and shoulders, place your hands closer together behind you and squeeze your shoulder blades together as you push your chest up. Imagine your head is a pitcher of water and you are pouring water out the top of your head as you arch back, and then returning the pitcher back to level without sloshing any water.

☯ *If the position of the hands hurts your wrists, try pointing your fingers to the sides. If you have a history of neck problems, don't arch the neck back; just look straight ahead.*

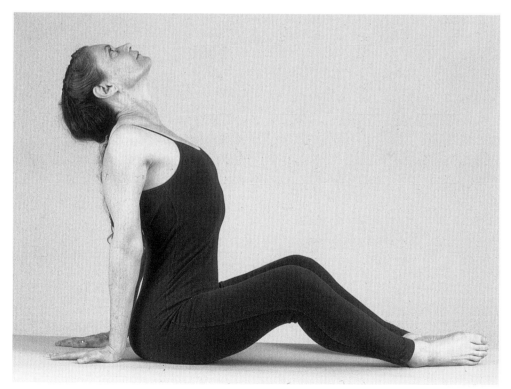

Photo 4.12

5. Pelvic Tilts

normal diaphragmatic breathing through the nose

Lie on your back with your knees bent and both feet flat on the floor, hip-width apart. Place your arms by your sides. You may place a folded towel under your head to help keep it from tilting back (photo 4.13).

Exhale and tilt your pubic bone up just enough to flatten the curve in your lower back (photo 4.14). Don't push your hips up or tuck so much that your tailbone curls off the floor. Then, inhale and tilt the pubic bone down, increasing the arch in your lower back (photo 4.15). Repeat 6 pelvic tilts both ways. Finish with imprinting the back in pelvic tilt with your belly hollowed out for 4 breath cycles.

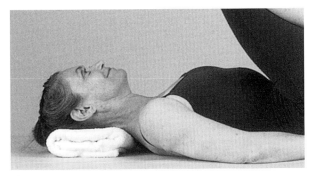

Photo 4.13

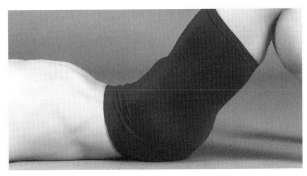

Photo 4.14

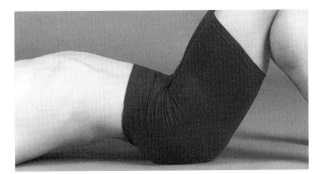

Photo 4.15

6. Single and Double Toe Touches

exhaling through the lips in the Pilates manner

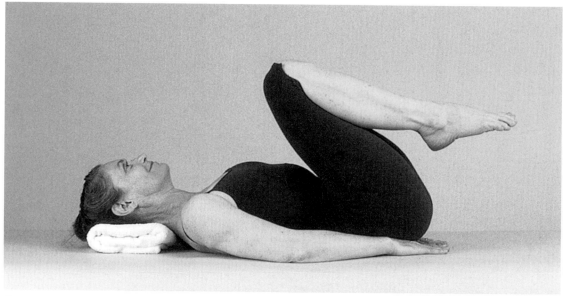

Photo 4.16

Lie on your back and bring your knees into your chest. Wedge your hands under the bottom edge of your hips to help you keep your back imprinted (photo 4.16). Leave your legs completely bent and relaxed as you exhale and lower one foot to touch the floor with your toes (photo 4.17). Keep your navel to your spine and control the action with your core muscles deep in your lower abdominal area. Inhale as you bring the foot back up. Repeat with the other leg, alternating toe touches slowly 6 times. Then, repeat 10 faster repetitions, lowering one foot as the other comes up. Keep an even pace with the breath, performing two touches for each inhalation and two for each exhalation.

Next, keep the legs together and fully bent as you exhale strongly and slowly lower both feet to touch the floor. Inhale as you bring them back up (photo 4.18). Use your core muscles and tilt your pubic bone up in opposition to the legs moving away, in order to keep the back flat and the stomach down. Repeat Double Toe Touches 5 times.

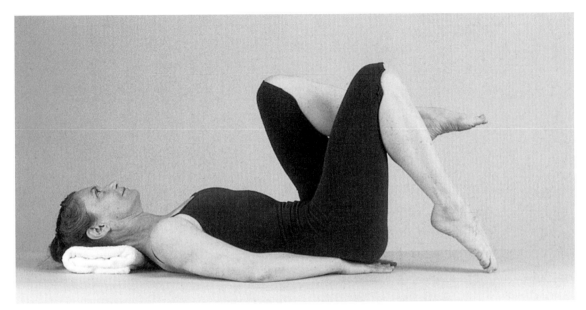

Photo 4.17

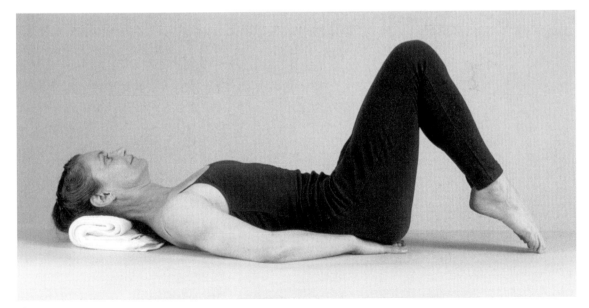

Photo 4.18

7. Slow Hundred

exhaling through the lips in the Pilates manner

Lie on your back with your legs together and bent 90 degrees in the air. Inhale and reach your arms straight to the ceiling without taking your shoulders off the ground (photo 4.19). Exhale as you curl up just to the bottom tips of your shoulder blades and push the arms down next to your sides (photo 4.20). Exhale all the air out of your chest, ribs, and lower stomach, and make sure the neck is in a long curve without pressing the chin into the chest. Your focus will be toward your knees, not the ceiling. Keep the belly deflated and the back imprinted, as you inhale lightly and raise the arms to knee height (photo 4.21). Exhale strongly as you push them back down. Maintain the position with your torso curled up and your legs in the air as you breathe with the arms up and down for 10 repetitions. Finish by lying flat with the knees into your chest.

As you get stronger, you can extend the legs straight to the ceiling as long as you can keep the lower back imprinted (photo 4.22).

☯ *If your neck gets tired or tight from curling up your head, you may do the exercise with the head down.*

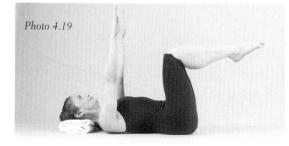

Photo 4.19

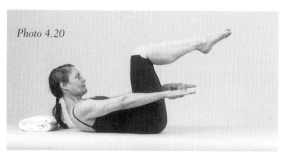

Photo 4.20

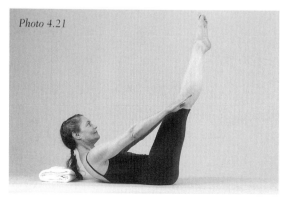

Photo 4.21

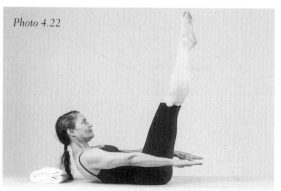

Photo 4.22

8. Leg Release

normal diaphragmatic breathing through the nose

Lie on your back and extend the left leg on the ground and hug your right knee into your chest. Make sure your thigh and lower leg are in a straight line, and not angled out or in. Also, be sure you don't hike up your right hip with the leg.

Relax the rest of your body as you circle the right foot 4 times in each direction to release the ankle joint (photo 4.23). Then, hold under the thigh and keep your calf and foot completely relaxed as you practice extending the leg up as you exhale and then back down as you inhale (photo 4.24). Repeat, gently extending the leg 4 times. Keep your thigh pulled in close to your chest and don't try to fully straighten the leg if it's tight. This is just a warm-up.

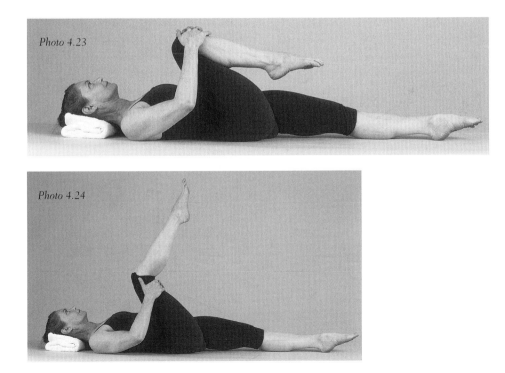

Photo 4.23

Photo 4.24

9. Single Leg Lift

exhaling through the lips in the Pilates manner

From your back, bend your left leg and place the foot flat on the floor. Rest your arms by your sides and extend your right leg up to the ceiling with the foot flexed (photo 4.25). Exhale as you slowly lower the leg toward the floor (photo 4.26). Inhale and lift the leg up again. Keep your belly hollowed out, the shoulders relaxed, and the pelvis in neutral. Repeat Single Leg Lift 5 times.

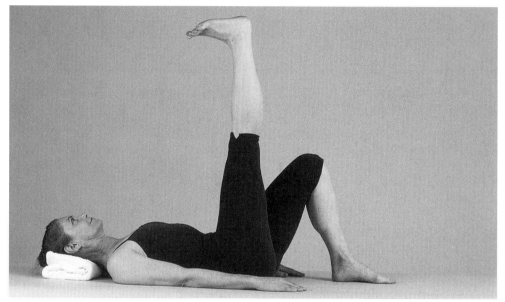

Photo 4.25

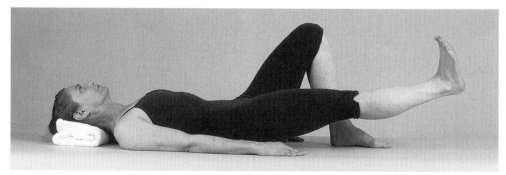

Photo 4.26

Single Leg Lift Variation

After you have practiced for a few weeks and you feel you are ready for a challenge, you may progress to this variation of Single Leg Lift.

Get some *light* dumbbells (2 or 3 pounds) and wrap a 3-pound ankle weight around your right ankle. Lie on your back with your right leg up, left leg bent, and hold the dumbbells next to your sides (photo 4.27). Inhale as you lower your leg and simultaneously lift the arms up parallel to your ears (photo 4.28). Exhale and bring the leg up and the arms back to your sides. Stay focused on keeping the pelvis in neutral, the leg straight, and your ribs and shoulders down. Repeat 5 times, then remove the ankle weight before proceeding to the next exercise.

Notice how when you reach your arms and legs away from your center, your core muscles have to work more to control them.

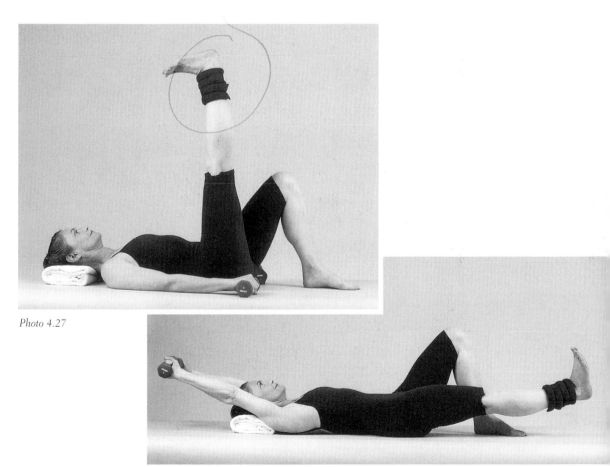

Photo 4.27

Photo 4.28

10. Leg Circles

exhaling through the lips in the Pilates manner

Lie on your back with the right leg straight up to the ceiling. Have the left leg bent with the foot flat on the floor, and your arms by your sides. Keeping your pelvis and shoulders anchored to the floor, circle the right leg counterclockwise, drawing an even circle in the air (photos 4.29, 4.30, 4.31). Inhale as you start the circle and exhale to finish. Pull your navel to your spine and think of your leg like a pen in a desk penholder that swivels around while the base holds still. Repeat 5 counterclockwise circles, finishing with the leg straight to the ceiling, and then reverse the circle 5 times.

☯ *If trying to keep the leg straight to the ceiling while keeping the hips down is too diffucult, bend the knee as much as needed so the hips stay flat and the thigh doesn't cramp up.*

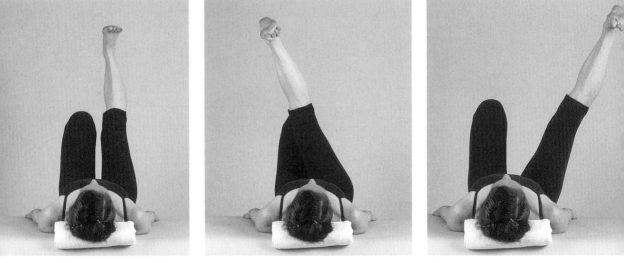

Photo 4.29   Photo 4.30   Photo 4.31

11. Leg Circle Finish

exhaling through the lips in the Pilates manner

From the ending position of leg circles with the right leg in the air and the left leg bent in, exhale as you curl up with your head and upper torso and grasp your right ankle (photo 4.32). Bend your right knee as much as you need to get to your ankle so you don't pull your middle back up off the floor. Inhale at the top and then exhale fully as you push your left leg out straight on the floor and pull the right leg in for a gentle stretch (photo 4.33). Keep your head and upper torso curled up until you complete the exhalation, and then inhale as you lower your head and release your right leg out on the floor.

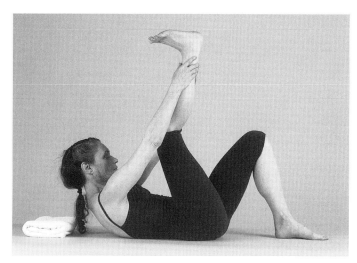

Photo 4.32

☯ *If reaching your ankle is impossible, grasp behind your knee instead.*

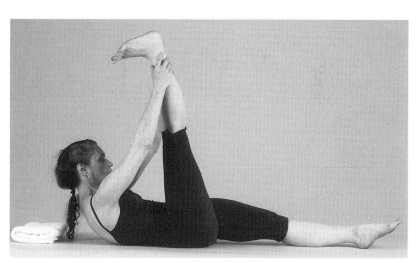

Photo 4.33

REPEAT EXERCISES 8–11 WITH YOUR LEFT LEG.

Note: Change the leg circle direction, starting clockwise for the first 5 circles.

12. Losing Your Breath ("Wind Relieving")

exhaling through the lips in the Pilates manner

Lie on your back and hold on to the backs of your knees (photo 4.34). Exhale as you curl up your head and upper torso and straighten both legs up, slightly less than a 90-degree angle from the floor (photo 4.35). Hold the legs lightly as you maintain this position, and exhale as much air as possible out of your chest, ribs, and lower stomach. This is called "wind relieving" and should take about 8 to 10 counts. At the end you will feel like you are losing your breath. When you have completely exhaled, relax your head down and bend the legs in as you inhale normally. Repeat this 3 more times. Be careful not to pull with your hands or round your middle back off the floor.

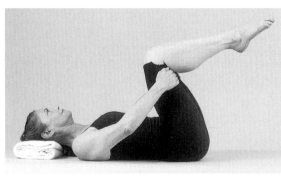

Photo 4.34

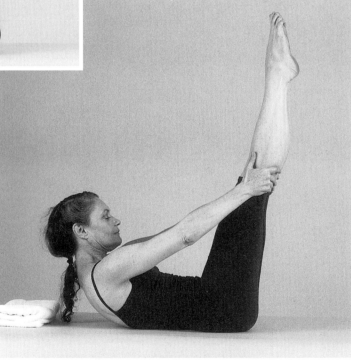

Photo 4.35

13. Single Leg Stretches
exhaling through the lips in the Pilates manner

Lie on your back with your knees bent into your chest. Exhale as you curl up with your head and upper torso. Lightly hold on to your right knee with both hands as you reach the left leg just below the 90-degree angle (photo 4.36). Keep your torso curled up and your back imprinted as you inhale and change legs. Then, exhale and change back. Repeat changing the legs 10 times, being careful not to let the outstretched leg drop down toward the ground. After a few weeks of practice, you can progress to reaching the outstretched leg to a 45-degree angle, as long as you can keep your back imprinted.

☯ *If your neck gets tired, you may place your hands behind your head, elbows to the sides, for support. And if you find it difficult to keep the back flat, alternate reaching the legs more toward the ceiling.*

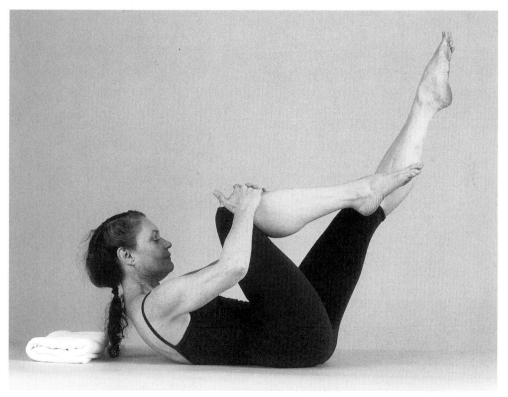

Photo 4.36

14. Open and Close

Ujjayi breathing through the nose

Lie on your back and extend your legs straight to the ceiling with your feet flexed (photo 4.37). To help keep the lower back imprinted, wedge your hands under the bottom edge of your hips. Inhale as you open the legs (photo 4.38). Exhale and close the legs back together. Repeat Open and Close exercise 10 times, emphasizing the exhalation from your lower stomach to power the closing of the legs.

❷ *If holding your legs straight up and your back flat is too difficult, bend your knees so your thighs can relax.*

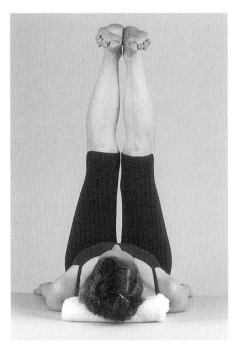

Photo 4.37

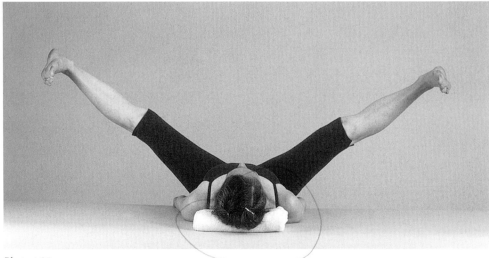

Photo 4.38

15. Walking with Pulses
Ujjayi breathing through the nose

Lie on your back and extend your legs straight to the ceiling with your feet flexed. To help keep your lower back imprinted, you may wedge your hands under the bottom edge of your hips. Inhale as you split the legs apart vertically to a normal walking distance (about 2 feet), and then exhale sharply as you stop the legs with a little pulse (photo 4.39). Inhale to switch the split and exhale again as you reach the stopping distance and pulse. Keep your stomach pulled in and your hips on the floor. Repeat 10 switches at a moderate tempo with distinct stops and pulses. As you become more practiced, you may increase the distance of the split between the legs.

☯ *If holding your legs straight up and keeping your back flat is too difficult,
bend your knees so your thighs can relax.*

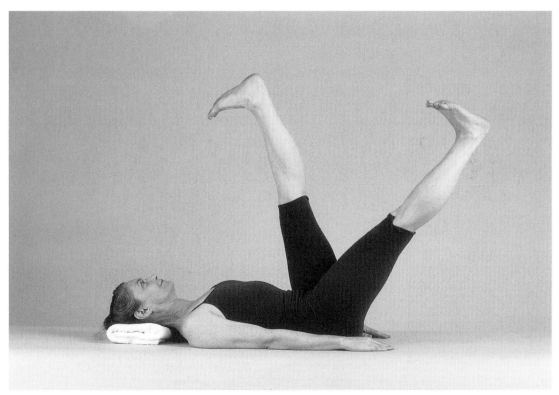

Photo 4.39

16. Knee Stirs

normal diaphragmatic breathing through the nose

Lie on your back and bend your knees
into your chest. Place your hands on
your knees and pull them apart and
around in opposite circles, releasing the
hip sockets. Relax everything as you
repeat 3 Knee Stirs one way and then 3
times the other way (photos 4.40 and
4.41). Finish by setting your feet on the
floor.

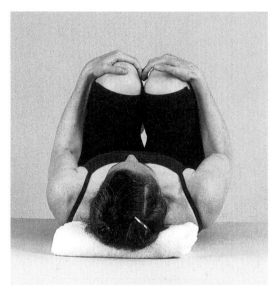

Photo 4.40

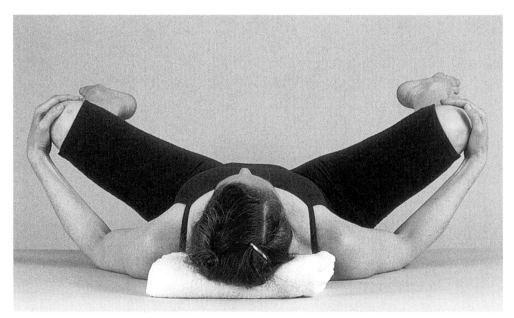

Photo 4.41

17. Pelvis Lift

normal diaphragmatic breathing through the nose

Lie on your back and bend your legs so your feet are flat on the ground, parallel, and hip-distance apart. Remove the towel from under your head and rest your arms by your sides. Exhale as you push with your feet to lift your pelvis off the floor (photo 4.42). Let your stomach, ribs, and chest relax down so you don't arch up your spine or push up with your belly. Walk your feet underneath your knees to where you can touch your heels with your finger. Keep your feet flat on the foor and concentrate on tucking up your pubic bone to feel a stretch in the front of your hips and thighs. Think of pulling yourself slightly forward with your feet to engage your hamstrings and buttocks. Take 4 full breaths in this position, and then exhale as you roll your spine back down from the top.

Repeat Pelvis Lift one more time, pressing up a little higher with your hips.

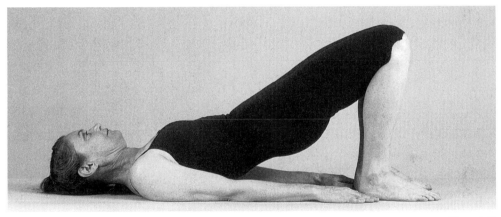

Photo 4.42

Transition from Exercise 17 to Exercise 18

On your back, exhale as you pull your knees into your chest with your hands and round up into a ball shape. Rock your body forward and back, rolling evenly along your rounded spine. Using your core muscles to help, rock yourself up to sitting.

❷ *If this is awkward, or too difficult a transition, simply roll to your side and then use your hands to push yourself up to sitting.*

18. Spine Stretch and Hip Hinge

normal diaphragmatic breathing through the nose

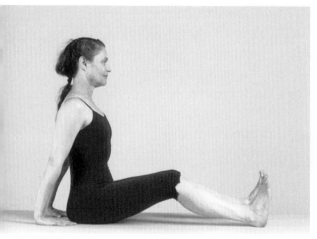

Photo 4.43

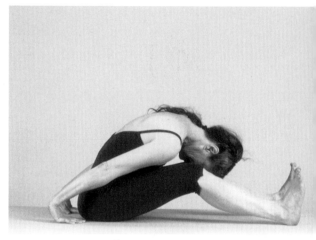

Photo 4.44

Sit up on the floor and open the legs just slightly wider than your hips (about 2 feet apart). Hold your legs in parallel, flex your feet, and allow your knees to bend slightly as you inhale and reach your spine up straight (photo 4.43).

Exhale as you round your spine over, curling from the top of the head toward the ground, but without tilting your pelvis forward (photo 4.44). Use your core muscles to round over and feel the stretch in your spine. Inhale as you roll your spine back up to sitting straight. Repeat one more time.

Next, exhale as you lean forward with a straight back, hinging forward from the base of your hips and pelvis (photo 4.45). You can press your hands into the floor to help brace up your back and push yourself forward. You should feel this stretch in the back of your legs. Inhale and bring your back up straight. Repeat forward hinge one more time.

As you become more flexible in your back and hamstrings, you can straighten your legs fully and reach forward with the arms for more stretch (photos 4.46 and 4.47). *Caution:* Do not grab your legs and pull, as this may injure your back.

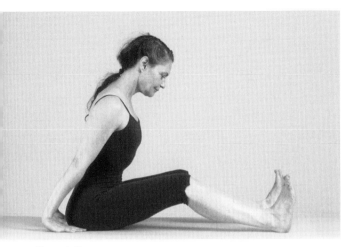

Photo 4.45

❷ *People with restriction in the hamstrings will find it difficult to sit up with the back straight. Place a firm pillow or folded blanket under your seat to elevate your hips and keep the knees bent, as in photo 4.2.*

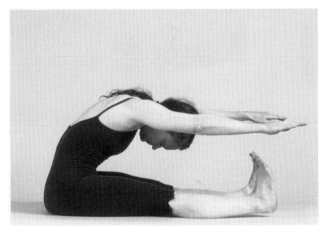

Photo 4.46

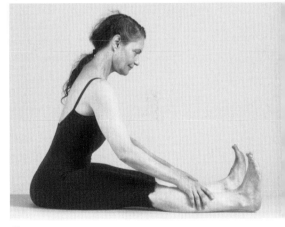

Photo 4.47

19. The Saw

normal diaphragmatic breathing through the nose

Sit up straight in the same position as in the previous exercise and reach your arms out to the side, palms down. Inhale and turn the top half of your torso to the right without twisting your hips out of alignment (photo 4.48). Exhale as you round over the right leg, pulling in the ribs and the navel, and reach the left arm down along the outside of the right leg (photo 4.49). Keep the spiral in your torso so your face and chest are facing the right side of the room, and don't let the legs come out of parallel with the feet flexed. Inhale as you lift to sitting up straight, and turn to repeat on the left side. Alternate sides as you do the Saw 3 times over each leg.

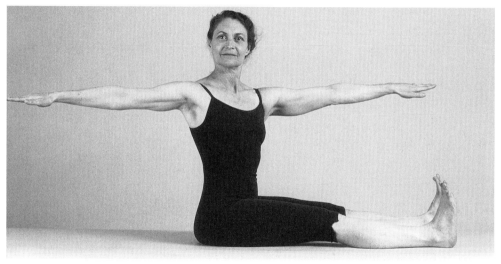

Photo 4.48

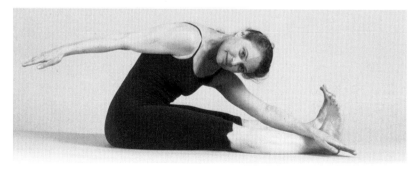

Photo 4.49

❷ *Again, people with restriction in the hamstrings should leave the knees bent and sit on a firm pillow.*

20. Single and Double Back Leg Lifts

normal diaphragmatic breathing through the nose

Lie flat on your stomach and place your hands under your forehead, elbows out to the side (photo 4.50). Feel the front of your body connected to the floor, particularly the front of your hips, and consciously lift your navel area up. Exhale as you lift one leg slightly off the ground (photo 4.51). Feel yourself reaching the leg out from under your hips, engaging your buttock muscles and core muscles, not the lower back. Keep the leg straight and make sure you don't lift the hip with the leg. Inhale and lower the leg, then repeat with the other leg. Alternate 5 Back Leg Lifts with each leg. Do these slowly to avoid gripping your leg or back muscles.

Then, exhale as you lift both legs off the floor (photo 4.52). Keep your legs parallel and close together. Again, you should feel this exercise in the buttocks and core muscles more than the lower back. Inhale as you lower the legs. Repeat Double Back Leg Lift 3 times.

❂ *If you feel your back tighten when trying to lift both legs, just do the single leg lifts.*

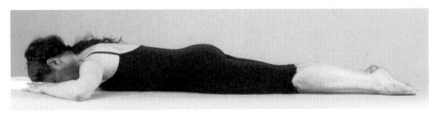

Photo 4.50

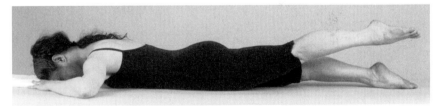

Photo 4.51

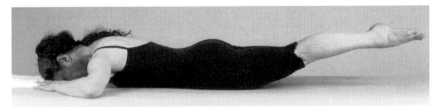

Photo 4.52

21. Sphinx and Supported Swan

normal diaphragmatic breathing through the nose

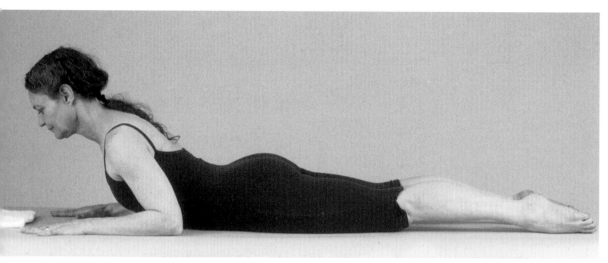

Photo 4.53

Lie on your stomach and place your hands level with your shoulders, elbows out to the sides. Press your hips forward into the floor, and inhale as you arch up the back. Rotate your elbows in under your chest, bringing the forearms in parallel, like a sphinx (photo 4.53). Keep your buttocks squeezed, belly in, neck straight, and pull your shoulders down. Exhale, open your elbows, and lower yourself back to flat on the floor. Repeat the arch to Sphinx 2 more times.

Next, lift to Sphinx one more time and then exhale as you push with your arms to lift up into a higher arch. Your arms won't fully straighten because you don't want to arch so high as to take the front of the pelvis off the ground (photo 4.54). Squeeze your buttocks, pull your stomach in, and keep your neck in line with your spine. Reach up through the top of your head as you inhale once in this Supported Swan position, and then exhale as you lower all the way down.

Note: Be careful not to arch the neck (photo 4.55).

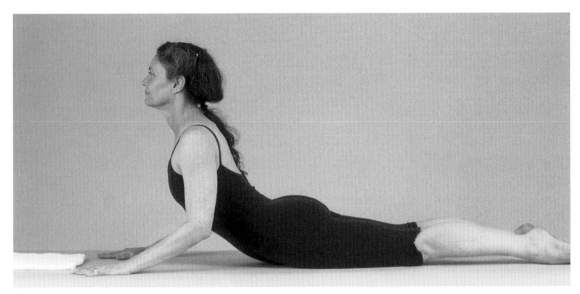

Photo 4.54

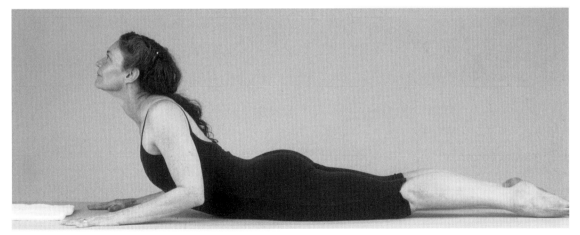

Photo 4.55

22. Child's Pose

normal diaphragmatic breathing through the nose

From your stomach, push your body back and fold over your legs (photo 4.56). Pull in your ribs and stretch your arms forward as you rest your head on the mat and your hips on your feet. Keep your legs parallel and close together. Take at least 5 slow breaths in this position and let the muscles in your back, shoulders, and hips completely relax.

☯ *If this position bothers your knees, place a soft pillow between your hips and feet.*

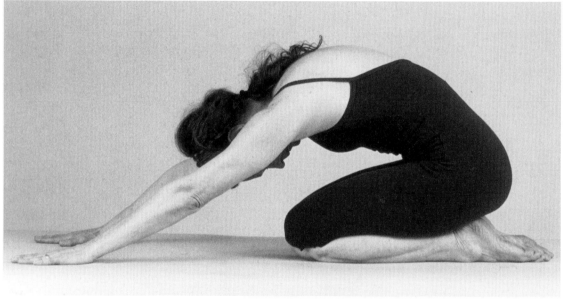

Photo 4.56

23. Cat Back

normal diaphragmatic breathing through the nose

Position yourself on your hands and knees with your back flat. Place the hands directly under your shoulders, fingers spread, and your knees under your hips (photo 4.57). Align the middle finger of each hand directly forward and keep your arms straight without locking the elbows.

Exhale deeply as you round your whole spine, head to tailbone (photo 4.58). Inhale deeply and reverse the spinal curve, arching it down as you reach the head and tailbone up (photo 4.59). Keep your shoulders down and arms straight as you repeat Cat Back 3 times.

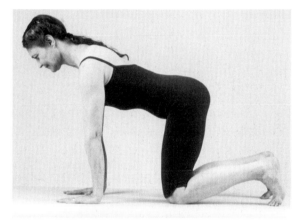

Photo 4.57

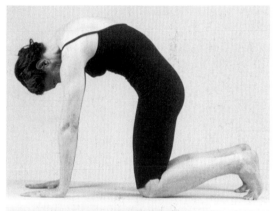

Photo 4.58

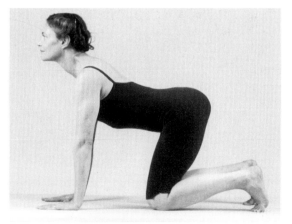

Photo 4.59

24. Downward-Facing Dog

Ujjayi breathing through the nose

From your hands and knees, with your back flat, walk the hands out about one hand distance forward from right under your shoulders, and curl your toes under (photo 4.60). Exhale as you push down with your feet, and raise your hips up to make an inverted V shape with your body (photo 4.61). Once your hips are all the way up, allow your heels to drop down toward the floor, feeling a stretch in the back of your legs. Keep your arms and legs straight without locking your elbows or knees, and feel your palms spread to distribute the weight evenly across all 10 fingers (photo 4.62).

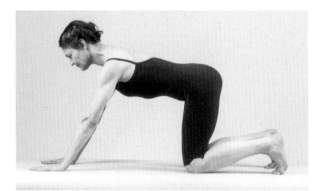

Photo 4.60

In Downward-Facing Dog, always work to keep your arms and back in one straight line. Resist pushing your ribs forward and feel the muscles under your arms connecting into the muscles along the sides of your back. Draw your shoulders down your back and rotate your elbows toward the floor without moving your hands. If you have a mirror, look and see if your neck and back are long and flat from your head to your tailbone. Keep your belly pulled in as you breathe strongly through your nose for 4 breath cycles. Finish by lifting up on your toes and bending your knees back to the floor.

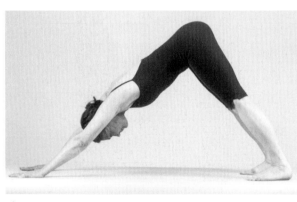

Photo 4.61

🌀 *If your lower back and pelvis are rounded, bend your knees to help release your back straight and tailbone up more. If it is still impossible to straighten your back in this position, go to a wall and practice Half-Downward-Facing Dog.*

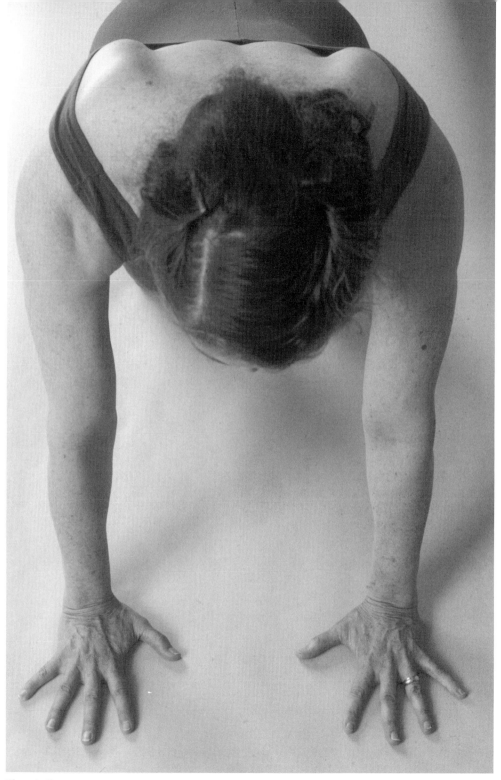

Photo 4.62

Half-Downward-Facing Dog

Stand half a body length away from the wall. Bend over from the hips 90 degrees, and place your hands on the wall (photo 4.63). Allow the knees to bend a little as you try to push your arms and back fully straight. Use a mirror to check yourself for correct form (photo 4.64). Work to get your legs straight with the heels reaching into the floor for 4 breath cycles.

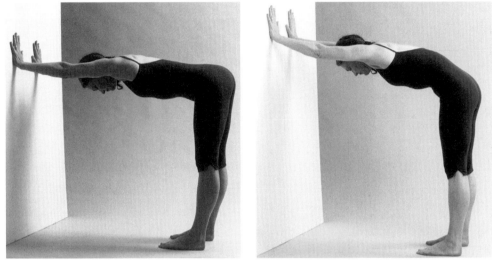

Photo 4.63   *Photo 4.64*

Downward-Facing Dog Variation

To help stretch your Achilles tendon in this position, place your feet close together and bend one knee as you press down the heel of the other leg (photo 4.65). Inhale as you lift up on the balls of your feet, then exhale as you change to stretch the other leg. Alternate legs 3 times. Then practice lifting both heels up with an inhalation and down with the exhalation 3 times. Your heels don't have to reach the ground (photo 4.66), and be careful not to lock (hyperextend) your knees. To finish, rise up on to the balls of your feet and lower back down to your knees.

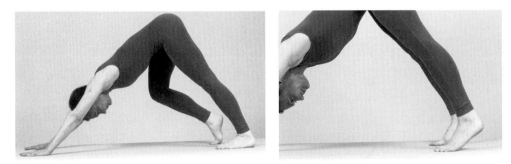

Photo 4.65   *Photo 4.66*

25. Rag Doll

normal diaphragmatic breathing through the nose

From your hands and knees, push your hips up and walk your hands back toward your feet to where you are hanging over your legs (photo 4.67). Your feet should be hip-distance apart and parallel. Keep your knees bent and allow your head and torso to hang freely. You can support some weight with your hands touching the floor or your shins. Feel your back and buttocks relax, pull your stomach and ribs in, and let your body fully fold in on itself. Don't sit your weight back on your heels as this makes the stretch less effective (photo 4.68). Relax in this position for 3 breath cycles.

When ready, release your hands from the floor or your shins, and hold your elbows, allowing the full weight of your torso, arms, and head to hang forward (photo 4.69). Completely relax your torso and just breathe with your diaphragm for 4 more breath cycles.

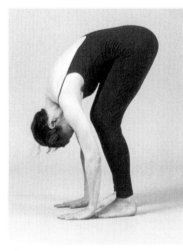

Photo 4.67

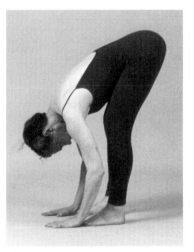

Photo 4.68

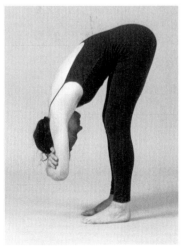

Photo 4.69

❷ *If you feel unsteady or uncomfortable in this position, you can put your hands on a foam block or footstool for added support.*

26. Flat Back

normal diaphragmatic breathing through the nose

From hanging over your legs in Rag Doll, place your hands on your thighs, bend deeper with your knees, and flatten your back parallel to the floor (90-degree flexion at the hips) (photo 4.70). Draw your shoulders down your back and feel the top of your head reaching forward as your tailbone reaches straight back. Feel your core muscles wrap around your lower torso for support.

Next, reach your arms straight back, parallel to your sides (photo 4.71). You should feel inherent power in this position, like a swimmer getting ready to dive into the water. Hold this Flat Back position for 4 breath cycles.

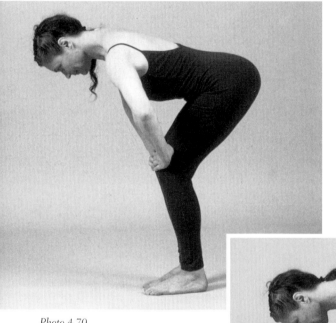

Photo 4.70

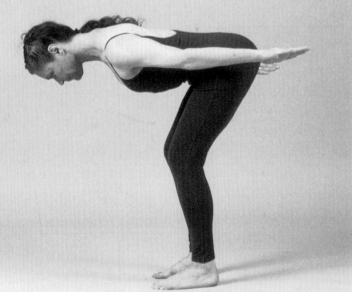

Photo 4.71

27. Standing in Neutral and Knee Bends

normal diaphragmatic breathing through the nose

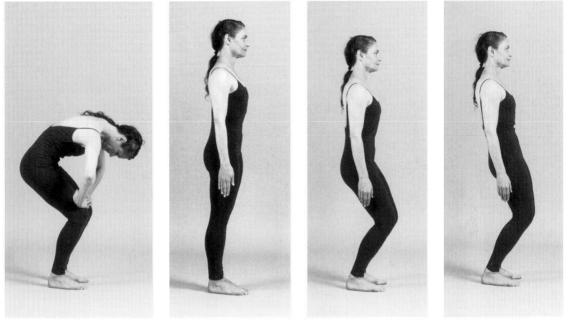

Photo 4.72   Photo 4.73   Photo 4.74   **correct**   Photo 4.75   **incorrect**

From Flat Back, place your hands back on the thighs and round up to standing (photos 4.72 and 4.73). Check your alignment, making sure your pelvis is neutral, your feet are parallel and hip-distance apart, and your knees are not locked straight (hyperextended). Feel your feet connected to the floor and your hips and buttocks relaxed.

Inhale into a small bend with the knees (photo 4.74), and then exhale as you straighten back up. Watch that you don't take your pelvis forward when you bend your knees (photo 4.75). Repeat 8 small Knee Bends.

28. Toe Raises and Balance

normal diaphragmatic breathing through the nose

From standing straight, exhale as you press down with the balls of your feet to rise up on your toes (photo 4.76). Watch that your weight doesn't shift toward your little toes as you rise up (photo 4.77). Keep the inside of your ankles in line with the big toes (photo 4.78). Inhale and lower back down. Repeat 8 Toe Raises.

Next, rise up on your toes one more time and balance. Float the arms up the sides and over your head without lifting the shoulders (photo 4.79). Stay up high on your toes and hold for 3 breath cycles. Then slowly lower the arms and your heels.

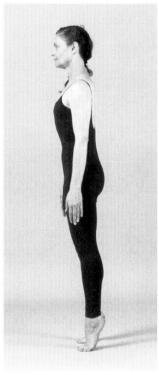

Photo 4.76

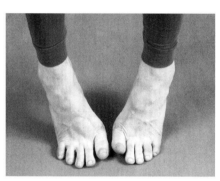

Photo 4.77   **incorrect**

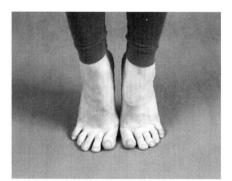

Photo 4.78   **correct**

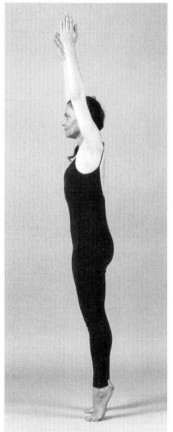

Photo 4.79

29. Tadasana: Standing Still and Tall Like a Mountain

normal diaphragmatic breathing through the nose

Place your feet together in parallel and your arms by your sides, palms facing in (photo 4.80). Lift and spread your toes out, and replace them on the ground, feeling a lift in your arches (photo 4.81). Release your weight into the floor by relaxing any tension in your lower back, hips, and buttocks. This will also allow the abdominals to pull in and the chest and shoulders to settle. Your pelvis should be hanging in neutral and you can visualize your tailbone dropping down like a plumb line toward your heels. Keep your chin level and your arms and legs reaching long. Practice standing still in Tadasana for 4 breath cycles.

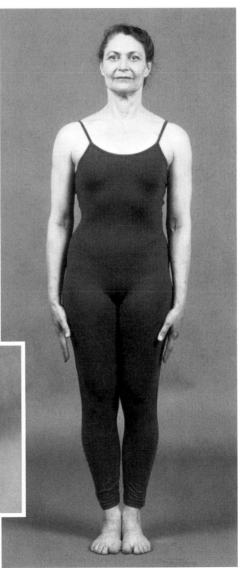

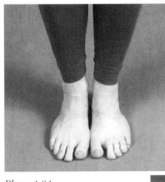

Photo 4.81

Photo 4.80

30. Modified Sun Salutation
Ujjayi breathing through the nose

1. Stand toward the front of your mat in Tadasana and bring your hands together in front of your chest (photo 4.82).

2. Inhale and reach your arms and face up, following the hands with your eyes (photo 4.83).

3. Exhale and swan-dive over the legs to a flat back (90-degree hinge from the hips) (photo 4.84).

4. Continue exhaling as you round your spine and bend the knees, placing your hands on the knees for support (photo 4.85).

5. Inhale and flatten out your back while keeping your knees bent (photo 4.86).

6. Exhale as you place your hands on the floor next to your feet, and then step both feet back into a push-up position (photo 4.87). Keep the hips up, level with your shoulders, and press your abdominals and ribs in for support. Inhale as you bend your knees to the floor.

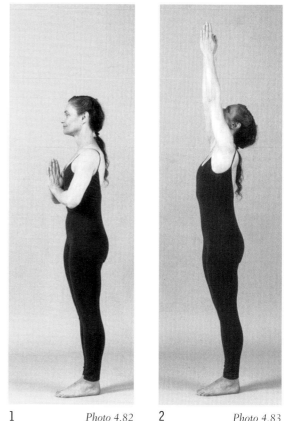

1   *Photo 4.82* 2   *Photo 4.83*

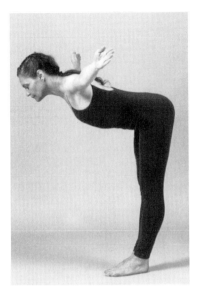

3   *Photo 4.84*

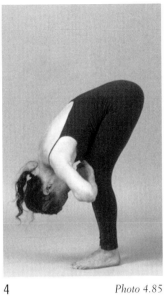

4   *Photo 4.85*

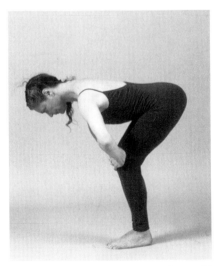

5   *Photo 4.86*

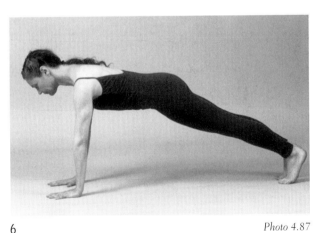

6   *Photo 4.87*

7. Exhale and bend your elbows to lower your chest to the floor (photo 4.88), and then place your stomach, hips, thighs, and forehead all flat on the floor.

8. Inhale and push yourself forward and up into Half-Cobra (photo 4.89).

9. Exhale, push back to your hands and knees (photo 4.90).

10. Then press up into Downward-Facing Dog (photo 4.91). Hold this position for 3 breath cycles, keeping your back flat, shoulders broad, belly in, and reaching your tailbone up and your heels down.

11. Inhale and bend your knees back to the floor (photo 4.92).

12. Exhale, step your feet together next to your hands, and fold your torso over your legs. Keep your knees bent and your hands touching the floor (photo 4.93).

13. Then, inhale as you place your hands on thighs and reach your back flat (90-degree hinge from the hips) (photo 4.94).

14. and 15. Exhale and reach your arms out to the sides and up as you stand up straight (photos 4.95 and 4.96).

16. Inhale and return to starting position with your hands in prayer (photo 4.97).

Repeat this salute to the sun, connecting all the movements with your breath and your core. Bring your arms to your sides and stand in Tadasana for 3 breath cycles.

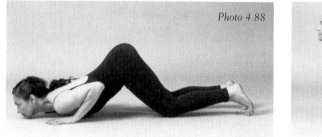

Photo 4.88

7

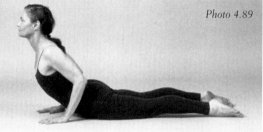

Photo 4.89

8

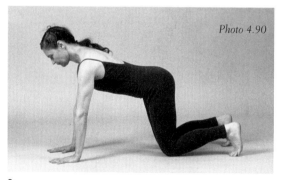

Photo 4.90

9

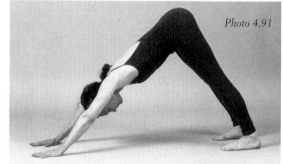

Photo 4.91

10

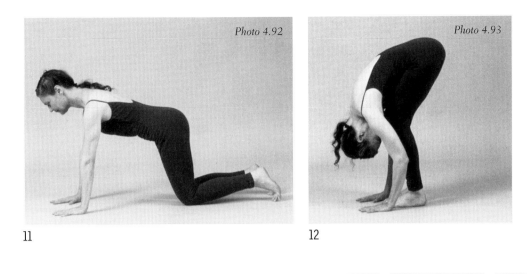

Photo 4.92

Photo 4.93

11

12

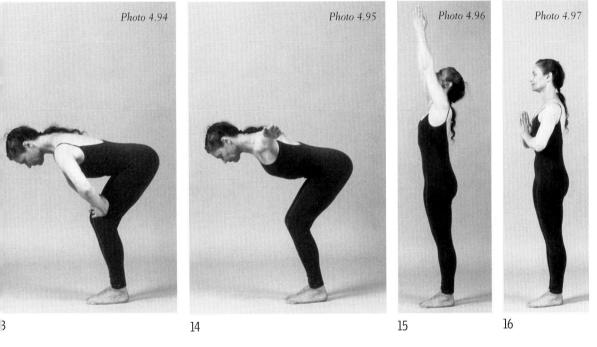

Photo 4.94

Photo 4.95

Photo 4.96

Photo 4.97

13

14

15

16

➋ *If supporting yourself in a push-up position is too difficult, just step back to your hands and knees, with your hands about 6 inches in front of your shoulders. Inhale in this position, and continue along.*

31. Chair Pose

Ujjayi breathing through the nose

From standing in Tadasana, inhale as you reach your arms down and up from the sides and bend your knees, sitting your hips back as if going to sit in a chair (photo 4.98). Press your legs together, keep your focus forward and your back straight. Sit back on your heels and see if you can lower your hips to where your legs are bent 90 degrees at the knee. Exhale and return to standing with your arms by your sides. Repeat Chair Pose 3 times, holding the last one for 3 breath cycles. Make sure you keep your ribs in, back flat, and the feet and legs together.

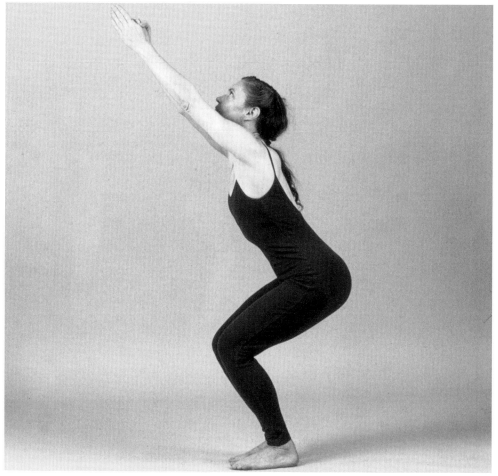

Photo 4.98

32. Supported Back Bend

normal diaphragmatic breathing through the nose

Stand with your feet hip-distance apart, neutral stance, and place your hands on your lower back. Inhale as you arch your spine backward, pressing on the hips with your hands for support (photo 4.99). Allow your legs to bend a little and your hips to move forward. Look up as you arch but don't drop the head all the way back. Exhale and return back to standing straight.

Repeat Supported Back Bend, this time keeping the legs straight and the hips in place, while still using the hands for support. This will isolate the stretch more in your abdominals.

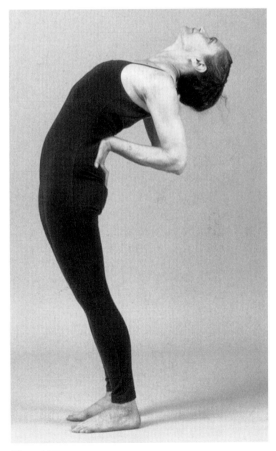

Photo 4.99

33. Warrior One

Ujjayi breathing through the nose

From standing with the legs together in Tadasana, place your hands on your hips and step your left leg back in a lunge appropriate for your height. Turn your left leg out from the hip about 30 degrees so that the sole of the left foot can be flat on the floor. Bend your right leg 90 degrees (photo 4.100), leaving the knee directly over the ankle, and keep the left leg straight. Keep the hips level and square to the front and settle your weight through your feet into the floor.

Inhale as you reach your arms up, palms facing in, and look toward your thumbs (photo 4.101). Exhale, place the hands together, and allow your elbows to bend so that you do not feel tension in your shoulders or neck (photo 4.102). Hold Warrior One for 3 more breath cycles feeling length and stability up and down your whole body. Then, lower your hands to your hips and step your left foot forward next to the right, back to Tadasana. Repeat Warrior One stepping the right leg back.

Guidelines for Establishing Appropriate Distance between Legs in Wide Stances	
In general, the distance between your feet in a lunge or wide stance in yoga positions is relative to your height.	
5'2"–5'7"	The feet are 3½–4 feet apart.
5'8"–6'1"	The feet are 4–4½ feet apart.
6'2"–6'7"	The feet are 4½–5 feet apart.
Use these guidelines for Warrior One, Warrior Two and Triangle Pose.	

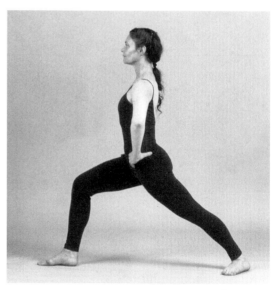

Photo 4.100

96

❷ *If reaching the arms up and looking
at the thumbs causes tension in your
shoulders or neck, bring the gaze forward
and lower the hands to your hips
(photo 4.100).*

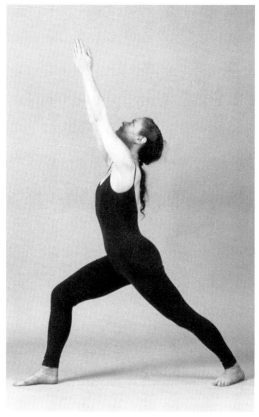

Photo 4.101

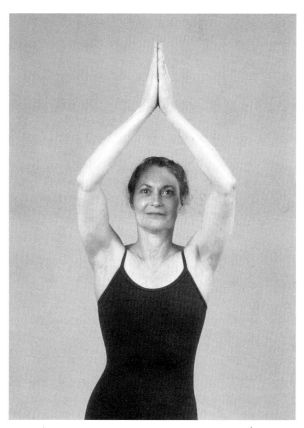

Photo 4.102

34. Warrior Two

Ujjayi breathing through the nose

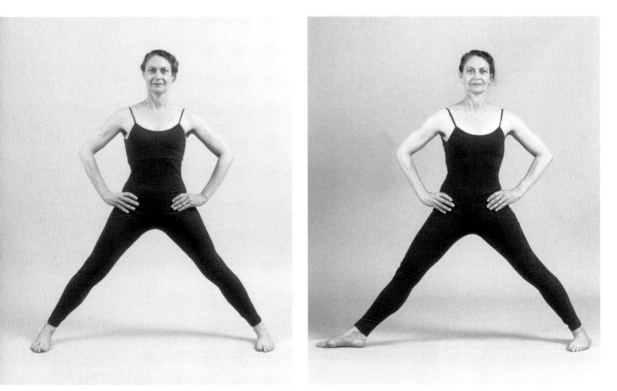

Photo 4.103   *Photo 4.104*

From standing with the feet together in Tadasana, turn sideways, and step your feet apart into a wide parallel stance (appropriate to your height) in the middle of your mat. Place your hands on your hips (photo 4.103). From there, rotate your right leg out 90 degrees to the right, and turn the left foot in 20 degrees (photo 4.104). Keep your hands on your hips so you can check to make sure your hips stay square to the front and don't dip down on the right side or tilt forward on the left. Feel your pubic bone reaching down and your tailbone under you to help keep your pelvis and spine straight.

Bend your right knee 90 degrees, keeping the knee directly over your ankle, reach your arms out to the sides and turn your face to the right (photo 4.105). Feel the connection between your legs and draw energy from the floor through your feet and up into your inner thighs and torso. Lift the inside of the left ankle so that it doesn't collapse in toward

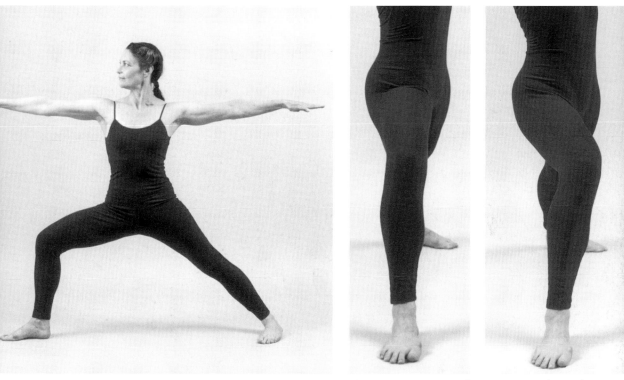

Photo 4.105   Photo 4.106   **correct**   *Photo 4.107*   **incorrect**

the floor, and check your right knee to make sure it stays in line with your foot (photo 4.106) and doesn't roll in (photo 4.107). Also make sure that the right knee doesn't extend past the toes. If this happens, it means your legs are too close together and you should place the left foot back a few more inches.

Hold Warrior Two for 4 to 5 breath cycles, stretching your arms long while the shoulders stay down. Then, face forward, place your hands on your hips, and turn both your legs parallel in the wide stance. Repeat Warrior Two on the other side. Finish by stepping your legs together in Tadasana.

☯ *If this pose bothers your knees, only bend the front knee 75 degrees. If you feel tension in your shoulders or neck, leave your hands on your hips instead of reaching them out.*

99

35. Triangle Pose

Ujjayi breathing through the nose

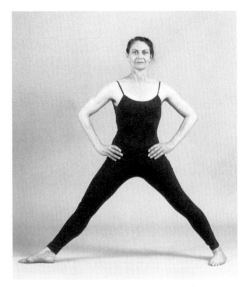

Photo 4.108

From standing in Tadasana facing sideways, step your feet apart to a wide parallel stance (appropriate to your height) in the middle of your mat and place your hands on your hips. Rotate your right leg and foot out 90 degrees to the right, and turn the left foot in 20 degrees (photo 4.108). Release your left hip out to the side and tilt the pelvis and torso over to the right, keeping your legs straight (photo 4.109). Be careful not to lock (hyperextend) your right knee, and don't arch your back.

The tilting of the body comes from the pelvis, not from curving over with the spine. Your sides should stay straight and your pelvis flat to the front. As in Warrior Two, don't let the back arch or the hips twist. The goal is not to see how far you can bend over to the side. It is to feel the straight geometry of the body as you actively stretch the legs and your torso.

Settle your weight evenly across the soles of your feet and wrap your core muscles around the torso for support. Extend the arms out, placing the right hand on the shin while the left reaches up to the ceiling (photo 4.110). Turn your gaze toward your left hand and hold this position for 3 to 5 breath cycles.

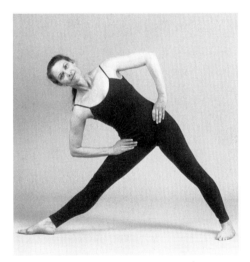

Photo 4.109

To come out of the pose, place your hands on your hips and exhale as you lift back up to standing straight. Turn the legs back to parallel in a wide stance. Repeat Triangle Pose to the other side. Finish by stepping the legs together in Tadasana.

❷ *If you feel tension in your neck or shoulders in this pose, keep your hands on the hips and the gaze forward as in photo 4.109.*

100

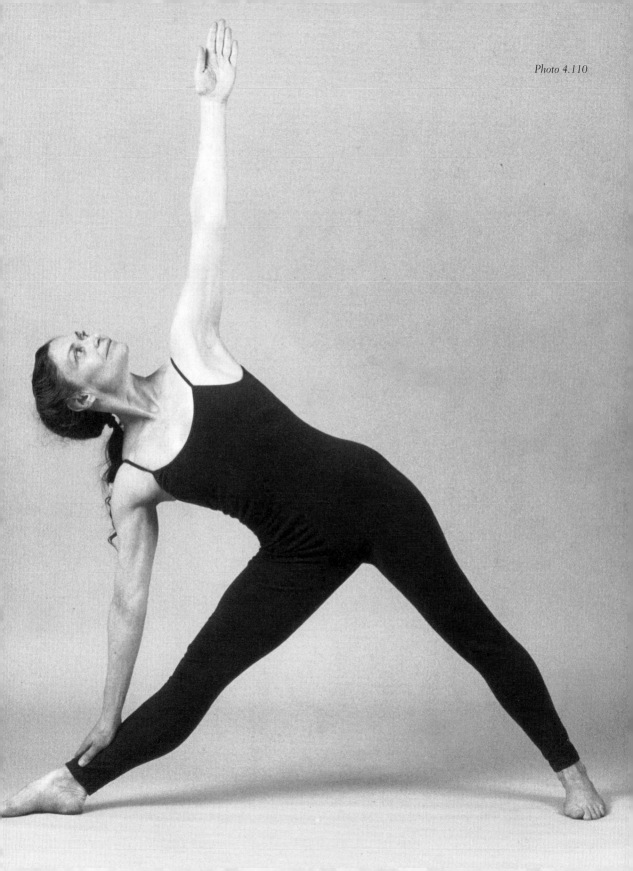

Photo 4.110

36. Knee Lifts and Tree Pose

normal diaphragmatic breathing through the nose

From standing with the legs together in Tadasana, exhale as you slowly lift the right knee up to hip height and inhale to set it down. Repeat lifting the right knee 3 times (photo 4.111). Think of this as standing knee folds, keeping the pelvis neutral and lifting the leg from the abdominals.

Next, exhale and lift the right knee one more time, turn the leg out, and place the sole of your right foot on the inside of your left calf (photo 4.112). Put your hands on your hips and balance for 3 breath cycles. Then, turn the right leg back to parallel and set the foot back on the floor. Repeat 3 knee lifts and the balance against the calf with the left leg.

Next, set the left foot down and lift the right knee up again. Turn it out and grab the ankle with your right hand. Lift the right foot up to place the sole of the right foot on the inner thigh of the left leg. Firm the muscles of your thigh as a brace against the fat. Keep the standing leg straight and maintain good alignment of your hips and spine. Feel the core muscles wrapping around the back and front of the torso and reach energy down the standing leg and up your spine. Reach your arms over your head with the hands together and balance in this Tree Pose (photo 4.113). Hold for 5 breath cycles, and then repeat on the other side.

☯ *If bringing the foot up to the inner thigh is difficult or makes you lose your balance, place it on the calf again for the second time as well. You can also keep your hands on the hips if reaching them up throws you off balance. Practice this until your balance feels steady before bringing the foot up and reaching the arms up.*

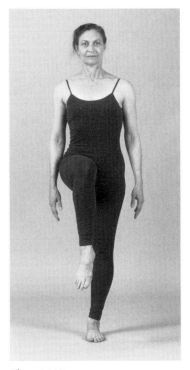

Photo 4.111

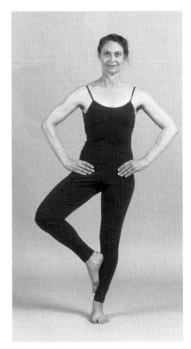

Photo 4.112

102

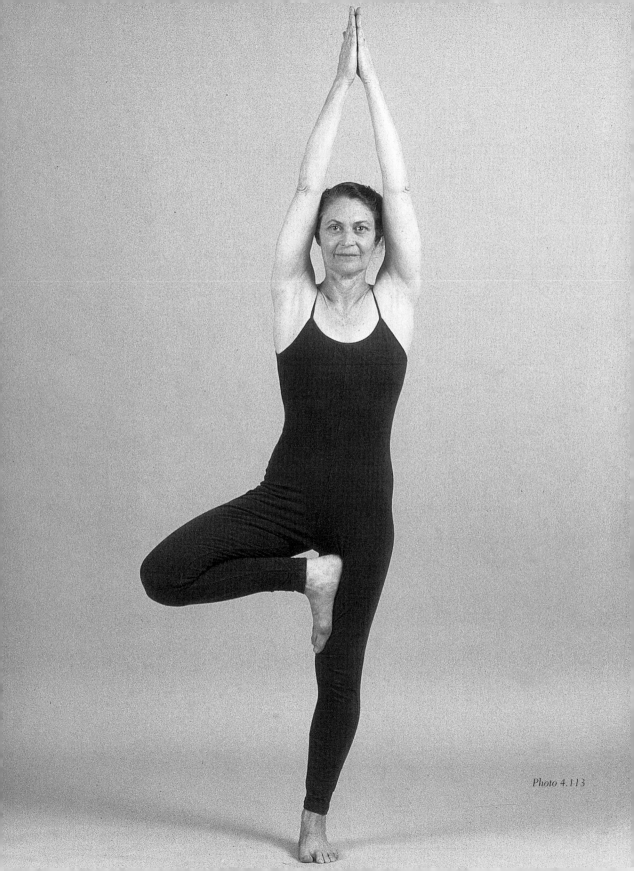

Photo 4.113

37. Seated Spiral

Ujjayi breathing through the nose

Sit on your mat, fold your left leg in, and cross your right leg over, bringing the right foot to the floor outside your left thigh. Hold onto your right knee with your left hand, and place the right hand on the ground behind you to support your straight back (photo 4.114). Keeping both hips on the floor, exhale as you spiral your torso around to the right, wrapping the left arm around the right knee (photo 4.115). Keep your back straight as you hold this pose for 5 full breath cycles, feeling the stretch in the right hip and buttock.

Unspiral the body and uncross the legs. Fold in your right leg and cross the left leg over the right. Repeat the Seated Spiral pose to the left side.

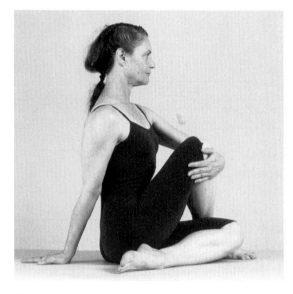

Photo 4.114

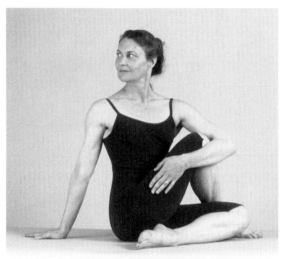

Photo 4.115

☯ *If folding the knee under you bothers the knee, stretch that leg out straight and then cross the other leg over before spiraling around (photo 4.116).*

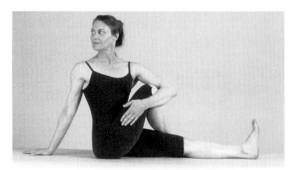

Photo 4.116

38. Half-Shoulder Stand and Easy Plow

normal diaphragmatic breathing through the nose

Lie down on your back with your arms by your sides and your knees bent into your chest (photo 4.117). Exhale and curl your hips up in the air and place your hands under them for support, bracing your arms on your elbows (photo 4.118). Keep your legs bent and hips balanced over your elbows. Draw your shoulders down your back and relax your neck and head. Hold this Half-Shoulder Stand position for 4 full breath cycles.

From Half-Shoulder Stand, allow the knees to come down toward your shoulders while leaving your hips back on your hands so the weight stays off the neck (photo 4.119). Your legs can partially straighten as you relax in this Easy Plow pose for 4 breath cycles. To come out of this pose, release your hands from your hips as you exhale and slowly roll down on to your back, keeping your legs relaxed. Engage your abdominals as you do this and press your arms into the floor for support. Finish on your back and bend your knees into your chest.

⚊ *If it is too difficult to lift the hips onto your hands or if it hurts your wrists, you can skip this exercise and just grab behind the knees and pull your legs and hips in toward your chest for a stretch on the lower back.*

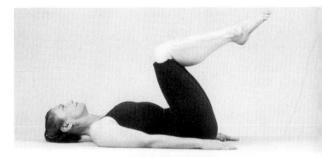

Photo 4.117

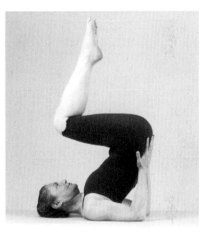

Photo 4.118

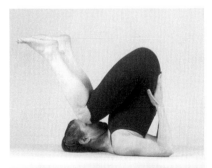

Photo 4.119

39. Shavasana: Full Release in Corpse Pose
normal diaphragmatic breathing through the nose

Lie flat on your back with your legs out straight on the floor. Place a folded towel under your head and relax your arms by your sides, palms up (photo 4.120). Close your eyes and completely let your body go. Even let control of your breathing go. Surrender your body to gravity and your mind to nothingness.

Stay in Corpse Pose for at least 3 to 5 minutes. When you're ready, bring the attention back to your breath, inhaling and exhaling deeply. Then bend your legs and roll over to your side in a fetal position. Enjoy the comfort and safety of this position for half a minute or so. From there, gently come up to sitting with the legs crossed.

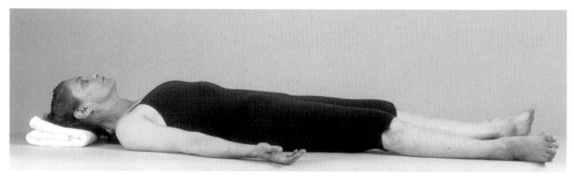

Photo 4.120

❷ *If it bothers your back to lie flat with the legs extended, or if you just want a more restorative position, place your legs up on a couch or ottoman (photo 4.121).*

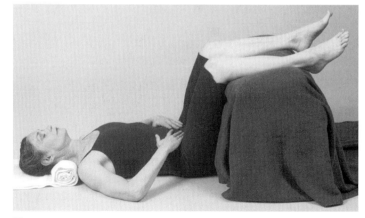

Photo 4.121

40. Meditation Pose

normal diaphragmatic breathing through the nose

Sit on a firm pillow or folded blanket with your legs crossed, and place the back of your hands on your knees (photo 4.122). Close your eyes and notice the ease with which you breathe and the stillness in the rest of your body. Feel yourself balanced with a long spine and neck, and let the muscles around your forehead, eyes, and jaw relax.

Imagine inhaling the air through the top of your head and down the front of your spine. Then, feel yourself exhale from your base up the back of your spine. Breathe slowly and effortlessly, feeling a sense of calm in your whole being.

To finish, place your hands in prayer position in front of your chest and bow your head. Feel your breath and let a soft smile happen behind your eyes and inside your mouth. Enjoy the peace and serenity of this pose as long as you want.

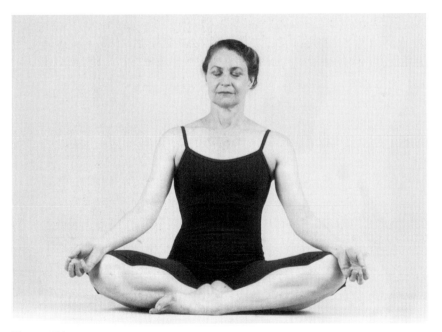

Photo 4.122

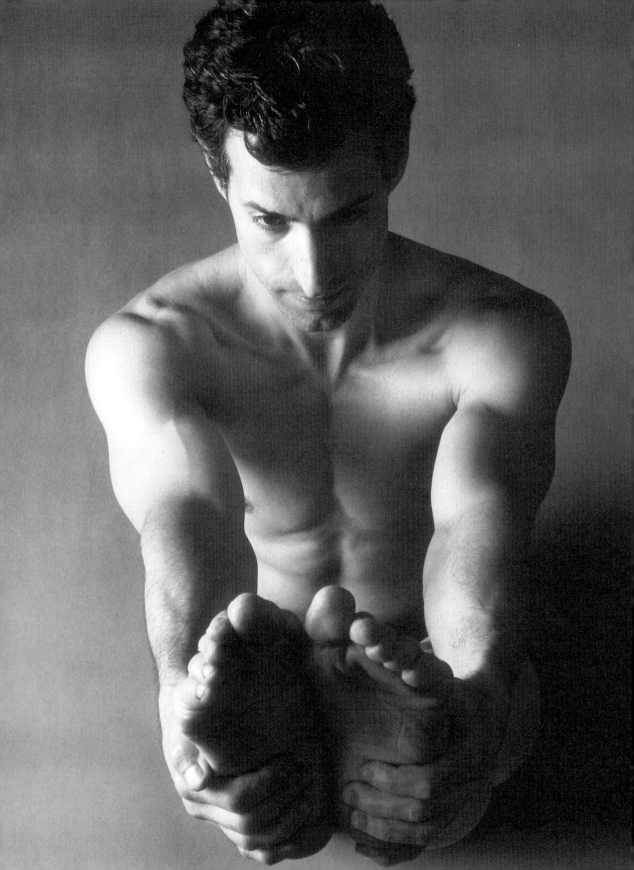

Chapter Five

Advancing Your Yogilates Practice

To be what we are, and to become what we are capable of becoming, is the only end of life.

—R. L. Stevenson

Advancing in your Yogilates practice is a great way to discover hidden talents, improve physical skills, and foster greater self-confidence. Diligent practice and an intuitive sense of your abilities will take you beyond old limits and into new heights of physical and spiritual satisfaction. But remember not to proceed in haste. Just because you have done all the exercises in the Beginner Series once doesn't mean you are ready to try the more advanced exercises. Assess your practice in terms of consistency, control, range of motion, ease of effort, and flow to determine your readiness for the next level. Remember that it is the quality of your effort, not the quantity of your poses, that equals success in your Yogilates practice.

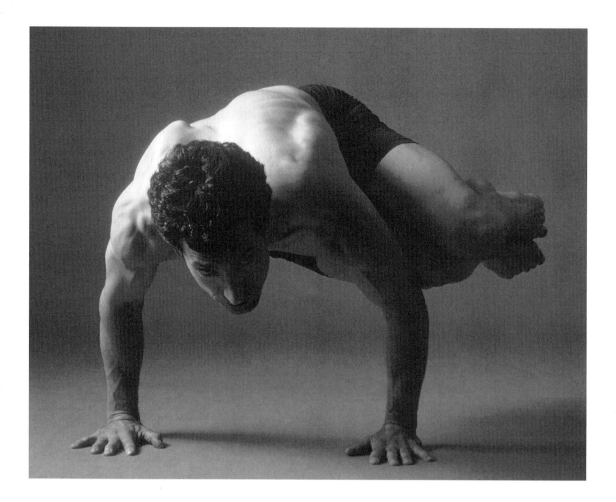

The exercise descriptions in this chapter include the focus areas of the body and how they relate directly to the earlier work. They are divided into two categories: Floor Work and Standing Exercises. Some are classic exercises from Pilates matwork or hatha yoga, some are unique Yogilates exercises, and some are simply more challenging versions of exercises previously described in Chapter 4. Sometimes exercises are linked together for greater efficiency and flow, although you should practice them individually at first. Expanding from the Beginner Series format, the earlier exercises are generally meant to go earlier in your routine and the later ones later. Remember always to start with breathing and warm-up exercises and to finish with Shavasana and Meditation.

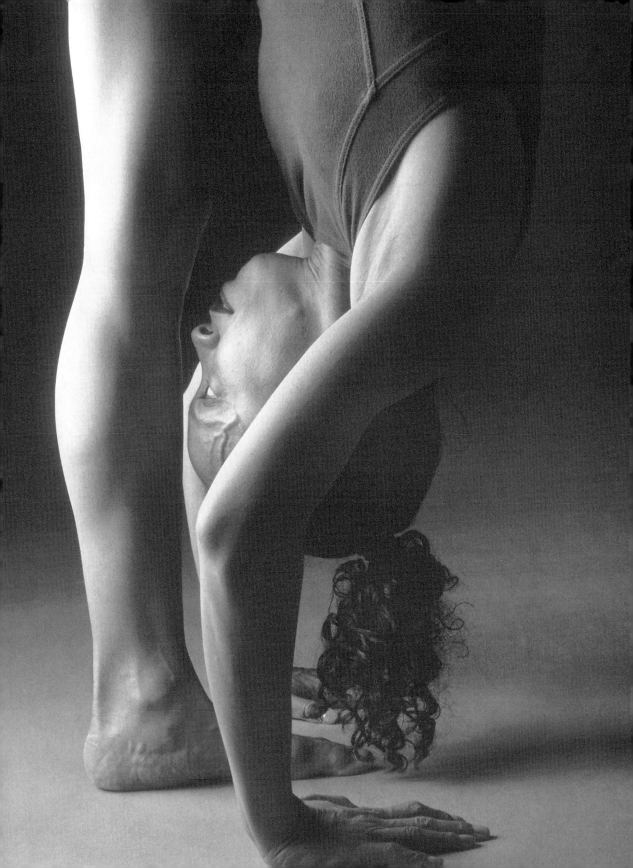

1. Half Roll-Downs with Twist

exhaling through the lips in the Pilates manner

Half Roll-Downs with Twist work your core abdominal muscles, tone your waist, and stretch your spine. This exercise would be substituted for Back Scoops, after Easy Pose and Arm Breaths.

Sit on your mat and bend both knees in parallel so the feet are flat on the floor. Place a soft 8-inch rubber ball or foam block between your knees (photo 5.1), and cross your arms at shoulder level (photo 5.2).

Press your knees against the ball, squeeze your buttocks, and exhale as you round your spine and roll halfway down to the floor, stopping before your lower back touches the floor (photo 5.3). Relax the head forward as you round your spine and tuck your pelvis. Then inhale as you roll back up to sitting straight. Repeat 3 Half Roll-Downs.

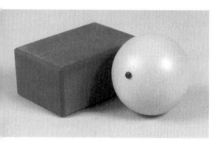

Photo 5.1

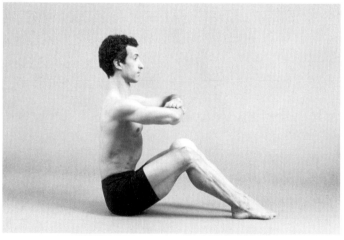

Photo 5.2

Next, from sitting straight up with your arms crossed at shoulder level, inhale and twist your torso to one side. Then, exhale as you roll halfway down, keeping the twist (photo 5.4). As you twist, squeeze the ball (or block) with your knees to help keep your hips square to the front. Notice if the ball (or block) shifts as you roll back. That will indicate that the hips are shifting as well.

Feel your obliques twisting your ribs and your lower abdominals pressing flat. Then inhale as you sit up straight again and twist to other side. Alternate 3 Half Roll-Downs with Twist to each side.

❸ *If you have a hard time keeping your feet on the floor when you roll halfway back, hook your feet under a couch to hold them in place. You can also make this exercise easier by crossing your arms over your stomach and only rolling back a quarter of the way.*

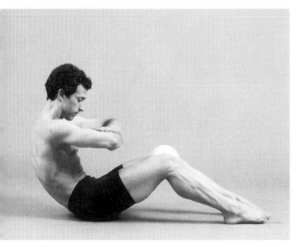

Photo 5.3

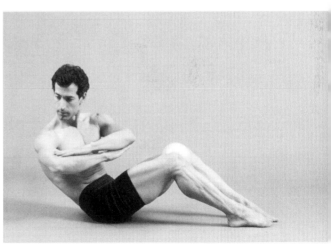

Photo 5.4

2. The Hundred

exhaling through the lips in the Pilates manner

The Hundred flattens the tummy, strengthens your core, and increases your circulation. This exercise substitutes for the Slow Hundred in the Beginner Series.

Lie flat on your back with your knees to your chest. Inhale as you reach your arms up to the ceiling, leaving your shoulders on the ground (photo 5.5).

Exhale fully as you push your arms down next to your sides and extend the legs out at a 45-degree angle. Curl up with your head and upper torso, leaving the middle and lower back imprinted (photo 5.6). Holding your legs still and torso curled, begin pumping your arms up and down in a small flutter.

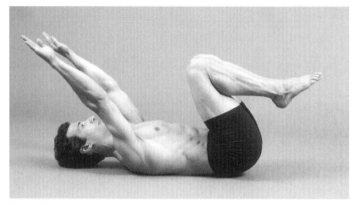

Photo 5.5

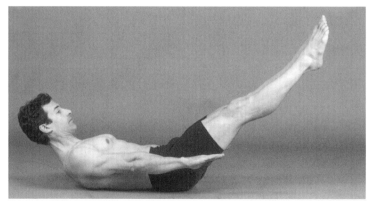

Photo 5.6

Breathe evenly over the pumping, inhaling for 5 pumps and exhaling for 5 pumps. Gaze at your knees and keep your belly hollowed, navel drawn to your spine. Pump the arms 100 times in this position.

As you become more practiced and your core muscles become stronger, you can do this exercise starting from lying flat and raising the legs up from the floor (photo 5.7 and 5.8) as long as you can keep your back imprinted.

☯ *If your neck gets tired or tight from curling your head up, you may do the exercise with the head down. If your thighs get tight, bend your knees to release the quads.*

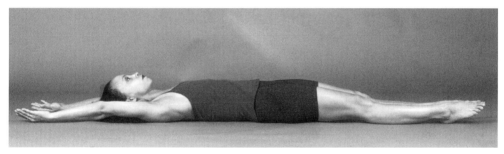

Photo 5.7

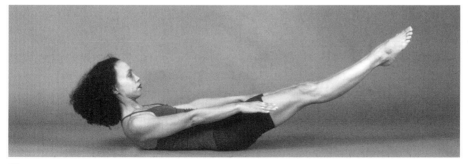

Photo 5.8

3. Bent and Straight Leg Roll-Ups

exhaling through the lips in the Pilates manner

Bent and Straight Leg Roll-Ups tone your abdominals and articulate and stretch your spine. This exercise traditionally would go after The Hundred. For greater challenge, perform all the roll-ups holding 2- or 3-pound dumbbells as shown.

Lie on your back with the knees bent and feet flat on the floor. Place a ball or foam block between your knees. Inhale as you lift your arms over your head, keeping the ribs

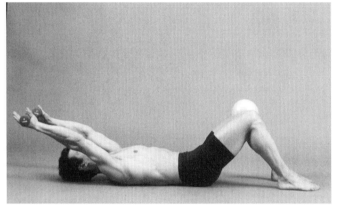

Photo 5.9

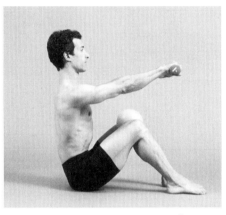

Photo 5.10

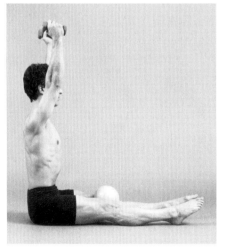

Photo 5.11

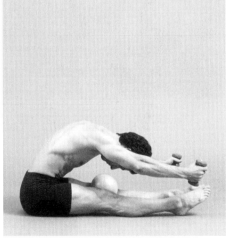

Photo 5.12

down and the shoulders drawing down the back. Exhale as you bring your arms forward and roll your body up to sitting straight (photos 5.9 and 5.10). Inhale at the top, and then exhale as you slowly roll back down. Try to roll down sequentially, vertebra by vertebra, reaching the arms forward until the lower back is flat. Repeat Bent Leg Roll-Ups 2 more times.

On the third roll-up, sit up straight, straighten your legs, and reach your arms overhead as you inhale (photo 5.11). Then exhale as you round your spine over your legs (photo 5.12). Keep the belly and ribs pulled in to maximize the stretch in your spine.

Inhale as you start rolling back halfway, keeping your back rounded and your arms reaching forward (photo 5.13). Then exhale, squeeze your buttocks, and tuck your pelvis as you finish the roll-down sequentially onto your back. Inhale and lift the arms over the head (photo 5.14), and repeat 2 more Straight Leg Roll-Ups.

☯ *If Straight Leg Roll-Ups are too difficult, you can practice only the Bent Leg Roll-Ups and hold the back of your thighs for assistance.*

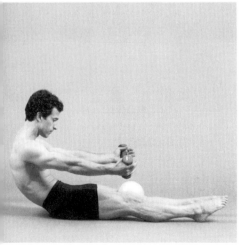

Photo 5.13

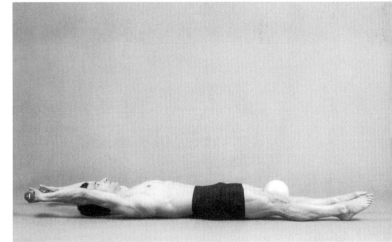

Photo 5.14

4. Rolling

normal diaphragmatic breathing through the nose

Rolling involves your abdominals, massages the back, and improves your sense of balance. This exercise traditionally goes after Leg Circles, although it can go anywhere in your floor workout.

From sitting up, hold on to your shins just above your ankles and pull your knees into you, lifting your feet off the ground and rounding your back as much as possible. Make a ball shape with your body, but be careful not to hunch your shoulders. Inhale as you roll back smoothly onto your shoulder blades (photos 5.15 and 5.16), and exhale as you roll forward to your buttocks. Avoid rolling so far back that you touch your head or so far forward that you touch the floor with your feet. Use your abdominals to stay in a tight ball as you roll back and forth 6 times, finishing balanced up on your seat.

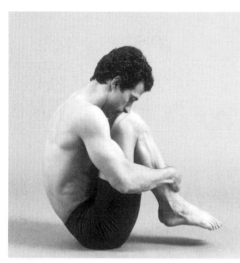
Photo 5.15

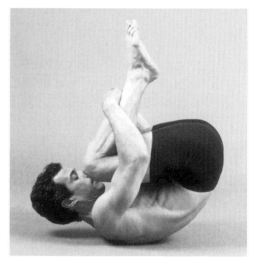
Photo 5.16

5. Single-Leg Stretches and Criss-Cross

exhaling through the lips in the Pilates manner

Single-Leg Stretches and Criss-Cross work your abdominals, with particular emphasis on your obliques. These exercises traditionally come after Rolling.

Lie flat on your back with your legs bent into your chest and your hands behind your head, elbows pointing out. Exhale as you curl up your head and upper torso and extend your left leg out at a 45-degree angle (photo 5.17). Make sure your back is imprinted and the belly is scooped out. Keep the head and shoulders up as you inhale and change legs, then exhale and change back. Repeat 8 Single-Leg Stretches, changing with each breath.

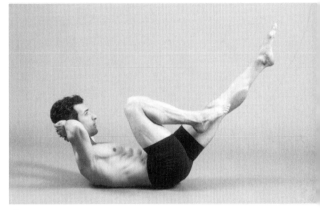

Photo 5.17

Then, double-time the leg motions to the breath, performing 2 leg changes for each inhale, and 2 with each exhale. Repeat 16 Single-Leg Stretches at this faster ryhthm.

Next, pause on the last leg stretch, with your right knee in, left leg out at a 45-degree angle. Exhale and twist your torso to the right, pointing your left elbow toward your right knee (photo 5.18). Keep your elbows wide and shoulders drawn down the back as you do the twist with your ribs, as opposed to reaching over just with the elbow. Staying up in your twist, inhale lightly, then exhale as you change legs and cross over to the other side. Repeat 8 Criss-Crosses, with a slight pause at the end of each one. Finish by lowering your head and torso and bringing both knees into your chest.

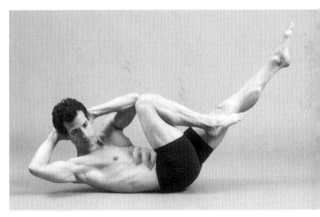

Photo 5.18

☯ *If this exercise is too difficult, do the Single-Leg Stretches as described in Chapter Four.*

6. Double-Leg Stretch

exhaling through the lips in the Pilates manner

Double-Leg Stretch strengthens your abdominals and inner rib cage muscles. This exercise would traditionally go right after the Single-Leg Stretches and Criss-Cross.

Lie flat on your back and hold your knees into your chest. Exhale and curl up your head and upper torso, leaving your middle and lower back imprinted (photo 5.19). Stay curled up as you inhale and reach your legs and arms out at 45-degree angles opposite each other (photo 5.20). Exhale as you bring your legs and arms back in. Make sure that your abdominals stay hollowed, ribs down, and back imprinted the whole time. Repeat 10 Double-Leg Stretches.

Finish by lowering your head and torso back to the mat with your knees into your chest.

❷ *If your neck feels strained while doing this exercise, you can place your hands behind your head and just move the legs. Also, if reaching the legs out to a 45-degree angle is too difficult, reach them straight up to the ceiling instead.*

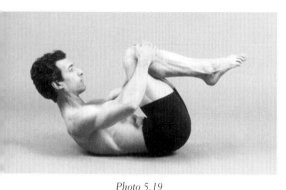

Photo 5.19

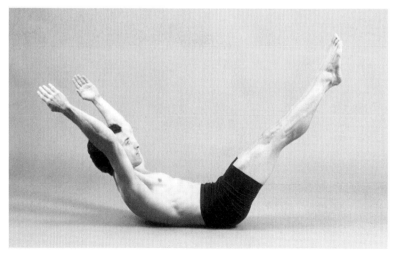

Photo 5.20

7. Scissors (aka Single Straight-Leg Stretch)

exhaling through the lips in the Pilates manner

Scissors strengthens your core abdominals and hip flexors. This exercise is normally placed after Double-Leg Stretch and can be substituted for Walking in the Beginner Series.

Lie flat on your back with your knees into your chest. Extend both legs straight to the ceiling. Exhale as you curl up the head and upper torso, and reach up to grasp your right ankle. Draw the right leg into you without lifting your hips, and lower the left leg to a 30-degree angle above the floor (photo 5.21). Keep your elbows pointing out and don't hunch your shoulders up.

Lightly do two short pulls on the right leg, then scissor-change your legs, and grasp the left ankle for two pulls (photo 5.21A). Inhale in the transition and exhale for the pulls. Keep your head up and back imprinted the whole time. Make the pulls small, focusing on the control of the legs from your core as you scissor. Repeat 10 Scissors with the legs. Finish by lowering your head and torso back to the mat with your knees into your chest.

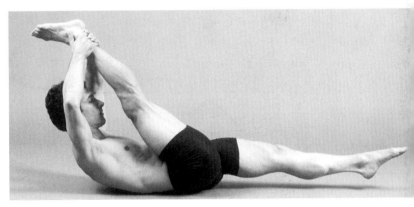

Photo 5.21

☯ *Make this exercise easier by allowing the legs to bend slightly and holding behind the knee. If your neck gets tired, place your hands behind your head for support and just move the legs.*

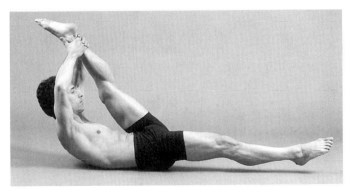

Photo 5.21A

121

8. Roll-Overs

exhaling through the lips in the Pilates manner

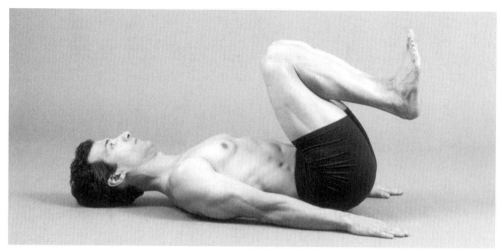

Photo 5.22

Roll-Overs work your lower and upper abdominals, the back of your arms, and articulate your spine. They also stretch the lower back. This exercise could be placed after Roll-Ups or after Scissors.

Lie on your back with your arms by your sides and your knees into your chest (photo 5.22). Inhale and reach your legs out to a 75-degree angle. Then exhale as you pull them in and roll back onto your shoulders with the legs over your head (photos 5.23 and 5.24). Pause with your legs parallel to the ground and your weight on the back of your shoulder blades, not your neck. Inhale here as you separate your legs hip-width apart.

Exhale as you slowly roll sequentially back down onto your back, keeping your legs close to your torso. Use your core muscles to control the motion and press your arms into the floor for support. As soon as your back is flat, bend the knees into your chest. Repeat 3 Roll-Overs, finishing on your back with the knees into your chest.

❸ *For less difficulty, extend the legs up to the ceiling instead of 75 degrees. You can also keep your legs bent during this exercise. If you feel a strain in your neck or back, skip this exercise.*

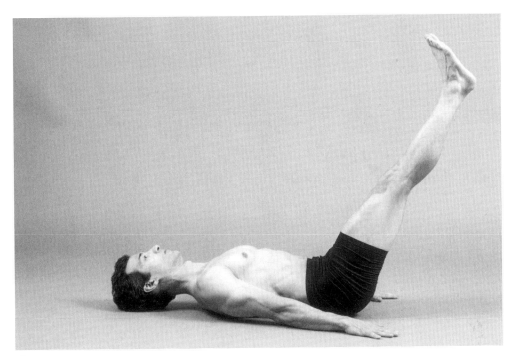

Photo 5.23

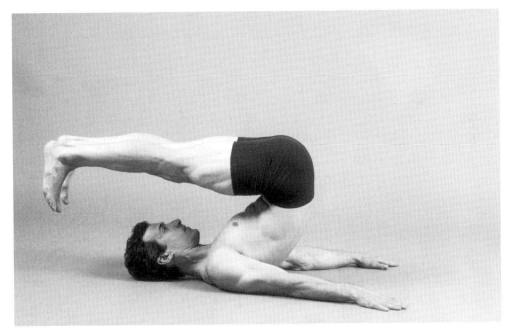

Photo 5.24

9. Fish Pose

Ujjayi breathing through the nose

Fish Pose stretches the front of your spine, chest, and neck. It also works your hip flexors and lower back muscles. This is a nice counterpose after Roll-Overs or Shoulder Stand, but it can be done anywhere in the floor part of your workout.

Lie on your back with your knees bent and feet on the floor. Push your hips off the floor and place your hands under them, palms down (photo 5.25). Set your hips down on your hands and extend your legs straight on the floor. Inhale as you push down with your elbows and arch up your spine, releasing your head back carefully (photo 5.26).

Try to get the top of your head to touch the ground without setting much weight on it. Hold Fish Pose for 3 to 5 breath cycles. To come out of this pose, exhale as you bring your head up and forward. Then push your body back off your hands to set your lower back on the floor. Rest flat on the floor for a moment, then hug your knees to your chest.

> ☯ *As an alternative to this exercise, sit up and place your hands behind your hips, fingers pointing to the back. Inhale and press down with your arms as you arch your upper spine forward, chest up, in Sternum Lift from the Beginner Series. Exhale to sitting up straight.*

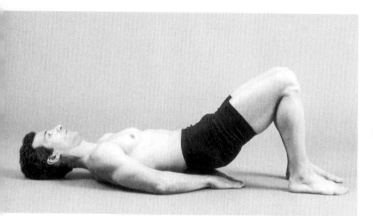

Photo 5.25

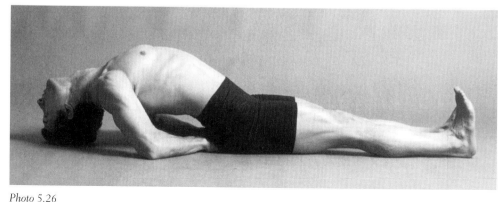

Photo 5.26

10. Bridge with Leg Lifts
exhaling through the lips in the Pilates manner

Bridge with Leg Lifts tones your buttocks and upper legs and stretches the hip flexors. This exercise could go after your abdominal exercises or after the Side-Lying Series.

Lie on your back with the knees bent, feet hip-distance apart, and flat on the floor. Exhale as you push your hips up and place your hands and elbows under them. Inhale as you reach one leg straight up to the ceiling (photo 5.27).

Exhale as you lower the leg to a few inches off the floor (photo 5.28), then inhale and lift it back up. You should feel a stretch in the front of the hip as you lower the leg. Perform 5 leg lifts and then repeat on the other side. Finish by lowering your hips back onto the floor and then gently pull your knees into your chest.

☯ *For less difficulty, lower the leg only halfway to the floor.*

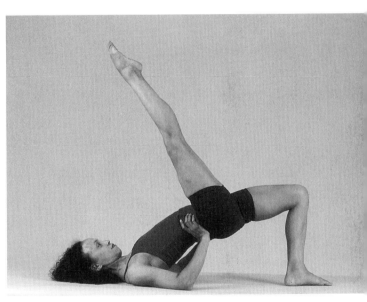

Photo 5.27

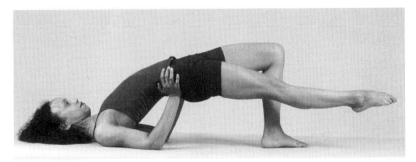

Photo 5.28

125

11. Teaser and Navasana

Ujjayi breathing through the nose

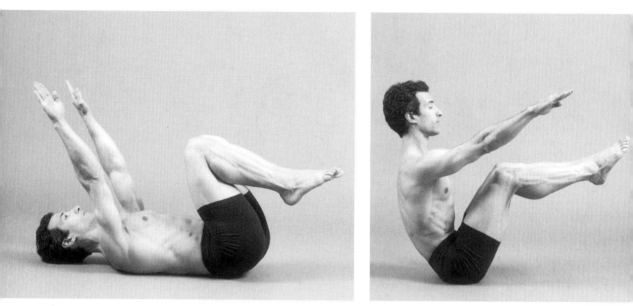

Photo 5.29

Photo 5.30

Teaser and Navasana strengthen and increase muscular endurance in your core muscles, and develop balance. These exercises could be placed after Fish Pose or Bridge with Leg Lifts, or they could go later in the floor routine after Side-Lying Series.

Lie on your back with your knees into your chest and your arms overhead (photo 5.29). Exhale as you bring your arms forward and curl up from the top of the head to sitting balanced up on your buttocks. Press your legs together in a 90-degree bent position (photo 5.30). Inhale in the balance, then exhale as you slowly roll back down on your back. Repeat 3 more Teaser curl-ups to balance.

On the last Teaser up, pause and see if you can straighten your legs at the top (photo 5.31). Then flex your feet, reach your arms parallel to the ground, and hold your balance

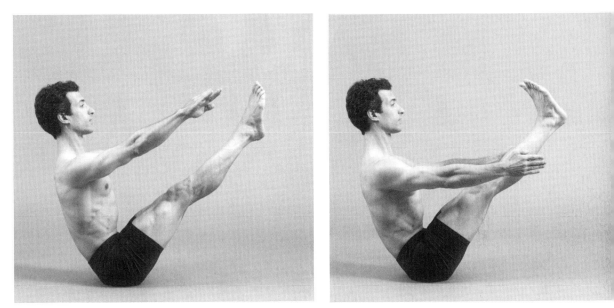

Photo 5.31   Photo 5.32

for 5 breath cycles (photo 5.32). This is called Navasana, or Boat Pose. Keep your navel pressed back to the spine, using primarily your core muscles to hold the legs in, not your hip flexors.

Finish by bending your knees and setting the feet on the ground as you sit up.

☯ *If straightening the legs in Navasana causes your thighs*
to cramp, keep your legs in a comfortable 90-degree bend.

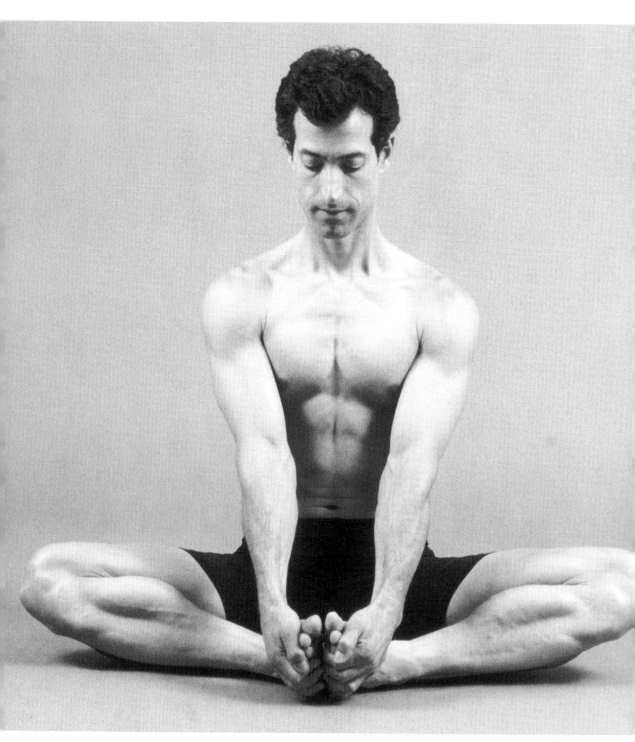

Photo 5.33

12. Cobbler's Pose

normal diaphragmatic breathing through the nose

Cobbler's Pose stretches your inner thighs and opens your hips. It can be placed after the exercises done on your back in the Floor Series.

Sit up and place the soles of your feet together, knees out to the sides, and use your hands to pull the feet in close to your hips (photo 5.33). Inhale and stretch your spine tall as you hold on to your feet and press your knees open. Then exhale and round your body forward (photo 5.34). Hold for 4 deep breaths, relaxing the back and inner thighs.

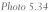 *For less difficulty, sit your hips up on a firm pillow and don't pull the feet in so close.*

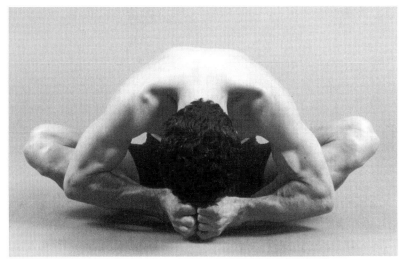

Photo 5.34

13. Straddle Stretch Lean and Head to Knee

Ujjayi breathing through the nose

Straddle Stretch Lean stretches and tones your inner thighs, and works your stabilization muscles. Head to Knee stretches your hamstrings and the sides of your lower back.

Sit on the floor and open your legs to a wide straddle, but not so wide that you feel a strain in your legs. Point your feet and brace your back up straight by placing your hands on the floor behind you (photo 5.35). Inhale as you reach up with the right arm, then exhale and lean over the left leg with a straight back (photo 5.36). Feel the back of your legs pressing into the floor, and keep your abdominals pulled in. Reach from your spine, not your arm, and keep both buttocks on the floor. Watch also that you don't arch your back or push the ribs out to the front. Inhale as you return to straight up. Alternate this stretch over each leg twice.

Next, flex your feet and twist your torso to face the left leg (photo 5.37). Keep your hips square to

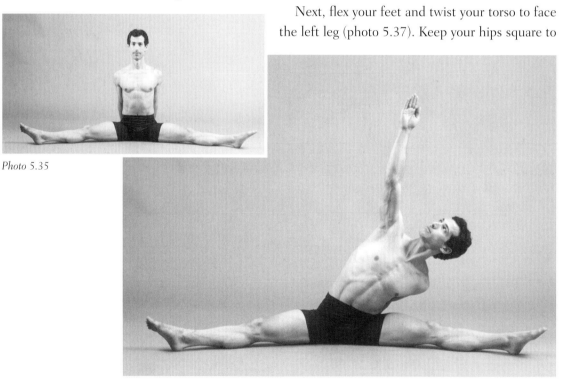

Photo 5.35

Photo 5.36

the front and exhale as you round over your left leg. Pull your abdominals in, let your head fall toward your knee, and reach your right hand to your left foot (photo 5.38). If you are flexible enough, reach around your back with your left hand and hold the side of your right hip. Hold this position for 3 to 5 deep breaths and feel the stretch in the back of your left leg and right side of your lower back. Exhale to lift back up and inhale as you twist to the other side. Repeat Head to Knee stretch to the left side.

☯ *If sitting on the floor with a straight back and your legs straddled is difficult, keep both hands on the floor for support and let your knees bend. You may also sit on a firm pillow or folded blanket.*

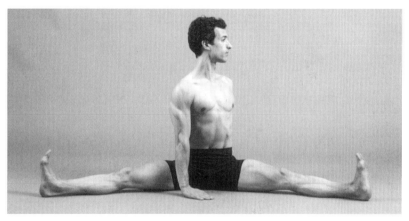

Photo 5.37

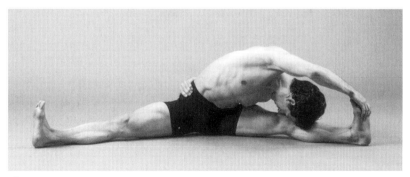

Photo 5.38

14. Reverse Plank and Forward Bend

Ujjayi breathing through the nose

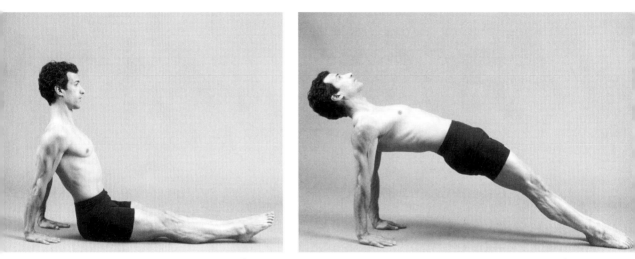

Photo 5.39

Photo 5.40

Reverse Plank tones the buttocks, lower back, and arms, and Forward Bend stretches the back of your legs and lower back. They can be performed after the Saw, or after Straddle Stretch Lean and Head to Knee exercises.

Sit with your legs extended out straight and place your hands on the floor behind you about 12 inches back, fingers pointing forward (photo 5.39). Lean back on your arms and inhale as you press your arms straight and chest up. Exhale as you point your feet and lift your pelvis up to bring your body into one straight line (photo 5.40). Hold for one full breath cycle, then lower your hips back down, and flex your feet. Exhale as you curve forward with your torso and stretch over your legs (photo 5.41). Take one full breath in this position, then sit back up straight.

Repeat, connecting Reverse Plank and Forward Bend with the breath 2 more times. Finish sitting up.

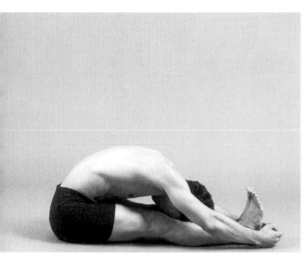

Photo 5.41

If pressing up to Reverse Plank with your legs straight is difficult, start with your knees bent and place your feet flat on the floor (photo 5.42). Then exhale as you press the hips and thighs up in line with the shoulders. This position is called Table Pose (photo 5.43). If your Forward Bend is difficult, you can sit on a firm pillow, allow the knees to bend a little, and keep your hands on the floor for support.

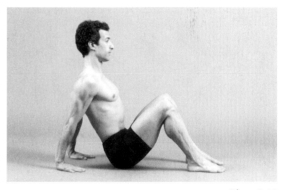

Photo 5.42

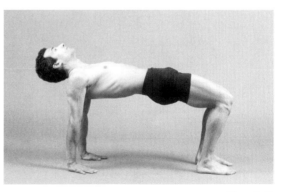

Photo 5.43

15. Runner's Stretch and Knee Balance

Ujjayi breathing through the nose

Runner's Stretch stretches your Achilles tendon, lower calves, and feet. Knee Balance strengthens your buttocks, lower back, and arms, and also develops balance. These exercises may go after Cat Back.

Position yourself on your hands and knees with your back straight and your arms straight and firm. Reach your left leg back, placing the ball of your foot on the mat (photo 5.44), and push your weight back toward your left heel to feel a stretch in the Achilles tendon and calf of your left leg. Hold this Runner's Stretch for 3 breath cycles.

Shift out of the heel to center your weight over your hands and knees. Exhale as you lift the left leg parallel to your torso, keeping your back flat and hips level. Then, inhale and reach your right arm forward and balance (photo 5.45). Keep your navel pressed back to your spine, your left arm straight, and your shoulders down as you hold Knee Balance for 3 breath cycles. Repeat these 2 positions on the other side.

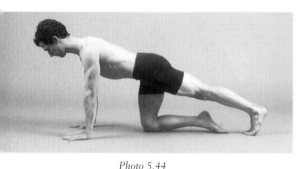

Photo 5.44

❷ *If your knees are sensitive, place a folded towel or a pillow under them.*

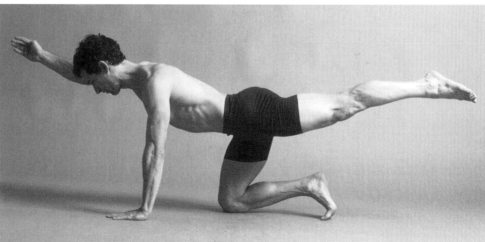

Photo 5.45

134

16. Forearm Plank

Ujjayi breathing through the nose

Forearm Plank strengthens and tones your chest and upper core muscles. It goes well after Cat Back or Knee Balance.

From your hands and knees, place your forearms parallel on the floor under your chest, shoulder-width apart (photo 5.46). Extend one leg back on the ball of the foot and then the other, and lower your hips to shoulder height as you hold your body in one straight line (photo 5.47). Pressing firmly into the floor, your elbows should be under your chest, and your face over your hands

Keep your navel pressed in, back flat, and feel the connection between your arms. Avoid letting your head drop or your shoulder blades pinch together. Hold Forearm Plank for 10 slow counts. Finish by bending your knees to the floor. Rest for 2 breath cycles, and then repeat for another 10 counts.

☯ *Modify by holding the pose for only 3 counts to start, working yourself up to 10 counts gradually.*

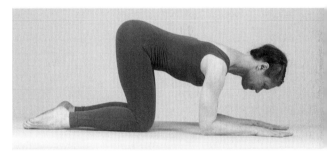

Photo 5.46

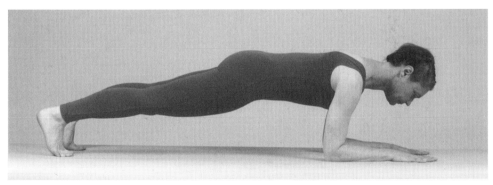

Photo 5.47

17. Swan to Swimming

Ujjayi breathing through the nose

Swan to Swimming strengthens and tones your buttocks and lower back muscles. It would go after Back Leg Lifts in the Beginner Series.

Lie on your stomach with your arms overhead and your legs together (photo 5.48). Inhale as you reach the arms behind you and arch up your torso (photo 5.49). Keep the legs on the floor and your neck in line with your spine. Exhale as you lower back down and reach the arms back over your head. Repeat lifting to Swan 3 times.

On the last lift to Swan, stay up with your torso and exhale as you reach your arms back around to the front and lift your legs off the floor (photo 5.50). Hold your body and legs

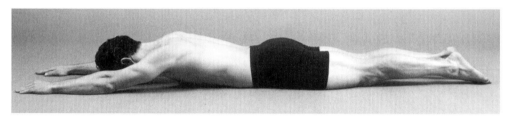

Photo 5.48

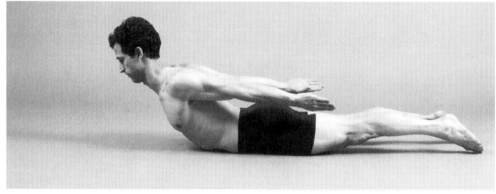

Photo 5.49

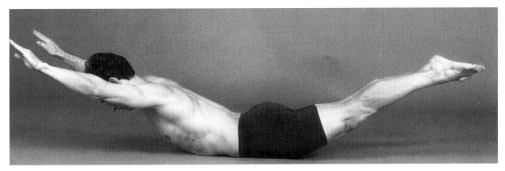

Photo 5.50

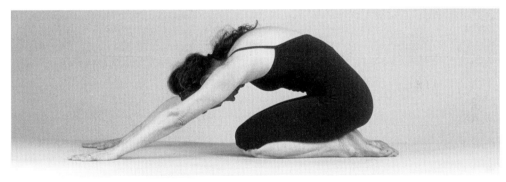

Photo 5.51

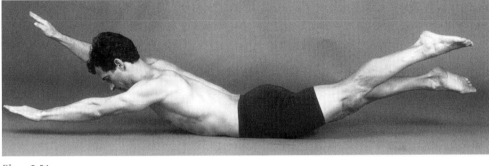

Photo 5.52

up as you start pumping the arms and legs up and down in opposition, as if you were swimming (photo 5.51). Inhale for 5 strokes and exhale for 5, for a total of 25 counts. Finish by exhaling as you lower everything down, and then gently push back into Child's Pose (photo 5.52).

☯ *If reaching your arms and legs up at the same time causes a strain in your lower back, skip Swimming and just do Single Back Leg Lifts.*

137

18. Bow Pose and Thigh Stretch

Ujjayi breathing through the nose

Bow Pose and Thigh Stretch stretches the chest, thighs, and front of your torso. It also strengthens and tones your back and buttocks. It goes in place of Swan and Swimming as a back extension exercise.

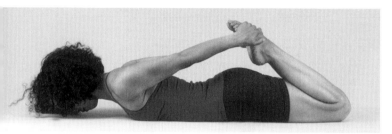

Photo 5.53

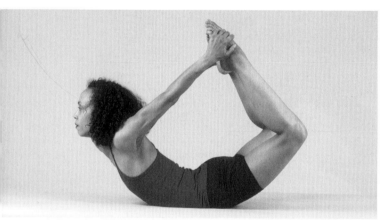

Photo 5.54

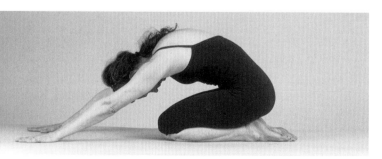

Photo 5.55

Lie on your stomach and bend your knees, bringing your heels toward your buttocks. Reach back with your hands and hold onto your feet (photo 5.53). Inhale as you lift up the torso and the legs into a bow position (photo 5.54). Press the feet out against your hands to help raise the legs, and allow your shoulder blades to pinch together to help stretch the chest. Hold Bow Pose for 1 to 2 breath cycles.

Exhale as you lower your torso and bent legs back down to the floor. Then, tuck your pubic bone forward as you pull your heels toward your buttocks for a stretch in the front of your thighs.

Repeat Bow Pose 2 more times, and then release your feet and push back into Child's Pose to stretch your lower back (photo 5.55).

☯ *For less difficulty, just do a Half Bow and Single Thigh Stretch. Hold onto one foot as you bow and stretch supporting yourself with the other hand on the floor. Then repeat on the other side.*

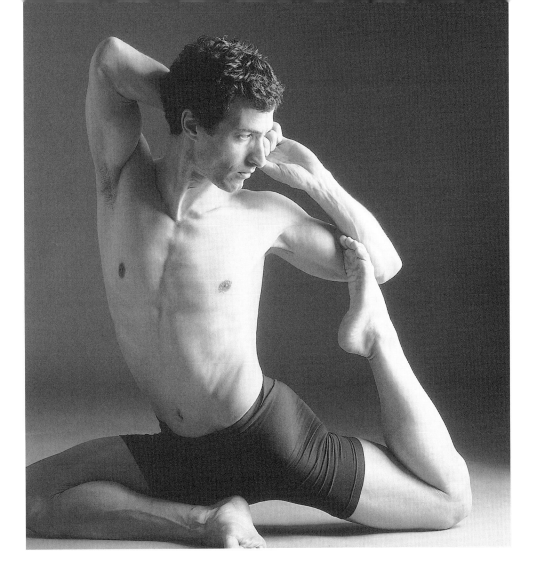

Side-Lying Series

The following 6 exercises tone the outer and inner parts of your legs and hips, and strengthen your side stabilization muscles. They fit into your routine after the back extension exercises on your stomach. Practice only the first 3 exercises for the first few weeks, and then add the following 3 to your routine. Perform them in order on one side of the body and then repeat the sequence on the other side. Make sure you have a thick yoga mat under the side of your hips to protect them from the floor.

19. Double-Side Leg Lifts

normal diaphragmatic breathing through the nose

Lie on your right side in a straight line, with your right arm overhead and your left hand on the mat in front of your stomach to help you balance. With your feet pointed softly, exhale and lift both legs together about 5 to 10 inches off the floor, being careful not to arch the back (photos 5.56 and 5.57). Inhale as you lower them back down. Repeat Double Side Leg Lifts 6 times.

On the last lift, hold the legs up straight, flex your feet, and bring your legs forward 30 degrees in front of your torso. Then, softly set them down. Keep your legs pressed together and your pelvis in line with your torso, as you hinge the legs forward from under your hips.

☯ *You can add support for your head by placing a rolled-up towel between your shoulder and the side of your head.*

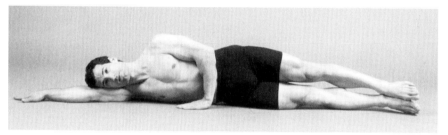

Photo 5.56

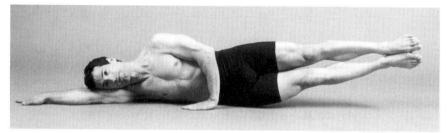

Photo 5.57

20. Side Leg Kicks

normal diaphragmatic breathing through the nose

Lie on your right side with the legs 30 degrees in front of your torso, feet flexed. Place your head up on your right hand and keep your left hand pressed into the floor in front of your stomach. Lift your left leg to hip height above the other leg (up about 5 to 6 inches) (photo 5.58). Keep both legs straight and hold everything in place with your core muscles. Exhale as you kick your left leg forward to about 90 degrees, adding a small kick or pulse at the end (photo 5.59). Inhale and point the foot as you smoothly sweep the leg back, slightly behind the line of your torso (photo 5.60).

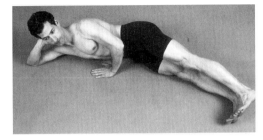

Photo 5.58

Focus on keeping your leg at hip height the whole time and your hips, torso, and shoulders perfectly still. Repeat 10 Side Leg Kicks, finishing with the legs together.

☯ *If you feel your hips or torso shifting around as you do the kicks, reduce the speed and range of motion of the kicks until you can control the motion.*

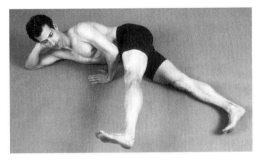

Photo 5.59

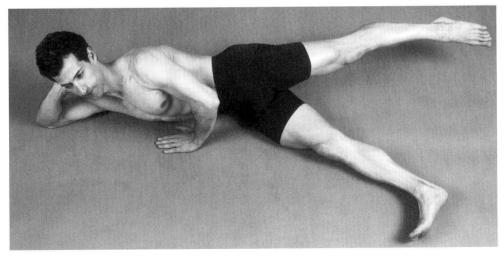

Photo 5.60

21. Side Leg Lift

normal diaphragmatic breathing through the nose

Lie on your right side with the legs 30 degrees in front of your torso, feet flexed. Inhale as you lift your left leg up to 45 degrees, keeping it parallel to the right leg with the foot flexed (photo 5.61). Exhale as you lower the leg with the foot pointed (photo 5.62). Make sure you keep your hips level and don't lift the leg with the side of your waist (hip-hiker muscles). Think of reaching your top leg out farther than the bottom leg and keeping your hips stacked over each other.

Repeat 5 Side Leg Lifts, flexing your foot as you lift and pointing as you lower, and then repeat 5 Side Leg Lifts, pointing your foot as your lift and flexing as your lower. Finish with the legs together.

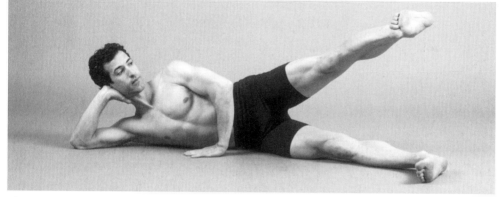

Photo 5.61

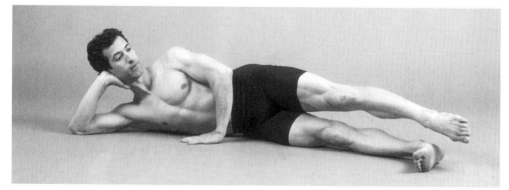

Photo 5.62

22. Inside Leg Lift

normal diaphragmatic breathing through the nose

Lie on your right side with the legs 30 degrees in front of your torso, feet flexed. Cross your left leg over the right, turning it out and placing your left foot on the floor in front of your right thigh. Hold on to your left ankle and be mindful not to tilt your hips back or round your back (photo 5.63). Exhale as you lift the right leg with the foot flexed (photo 5.64), inhale, as you lower. Repeat 10 Inside Leg Lifts, using your inner thigh and core abdominals to lift the leg back.

☯ *If placing your left foot on the floor is too difficult because of tightness*
in your hips, lift the left knee up in parallel to hip height and place it on the floor.
Place your hand on the floor in front and then proceed with the exercise.

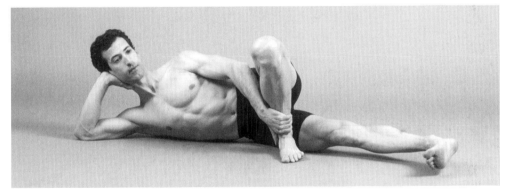

Photo 5.63

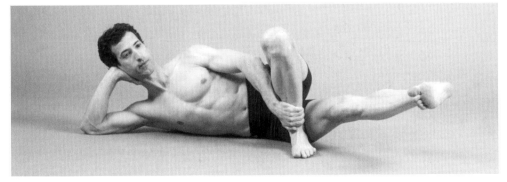

Photo 5.64

23. Open and Close and Turn-Out Stretch

normal diaphragmatic breathing through the nose

Lie on your right side with the legs 30 degrees in front of your torso, feet flexed. Bend your knees and bring them to hip height, as if you were sitting in a chair. Inhale as you rotate your left thigh open as far as you can without tilting the hip back, and point your left toes to the inside of your right ankle (photo 5.65). Exhale as you turn your left thigh all the way in (photo 5.66). Repeat Open and Closes 10 times.

Next, open your left thigh one more time and reach down with your left hand and grab your left heel (photo 5.67). Exhale as you straighten your left leg up and also push the right leg down straight (photo 5.68). Turn out both legs, flex your left foot, and pull the leg into you. Breathe into Turn-Out Stretch for 2 breath cycles. Finish by releasing the left heel, place your left hand on the floor in front of you, and then slowly lower your left leg straight down onto the right, keeping both legs stretched long.

❷ *If holding on to your heel in the stretch is too difficult, hold on to your calf instead.*

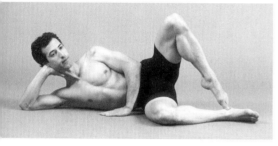

Photo 5.65

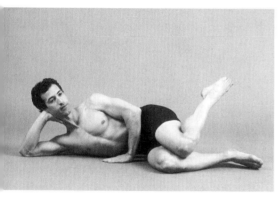

Photo 5.66

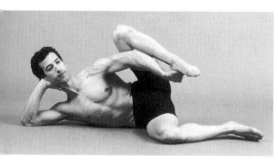

Photo 5.67

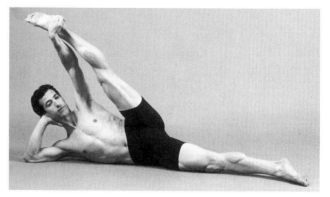

Photo 5.68

24. Heel Beats and Flutter Kicks
normal diaphragmatic breathing through the nose

Lie on your right side with the legs 30 degrees in front of your torso, feet pointed, and both legs turned out. Exhale as you lift them 6 inches above the floor with the heels and inner thighs pressed together (photo 5.69). Quickly open and close the legs, separating the feet only 2 to 3 inches apart, beating the heels together 20 times.

Next, keep your legs suspended in the air and rotate the legs back to parallel. Then quickly flutter-kick with your legs 20 times (photo 5.70). Hold your body stable as you move the legs from your center. Finish with the legs together and lower them to the floor.

☯ *If moving the legs quickly throws your balance off, move the legs slower for only 10 beats and 10 flutter kicks.*

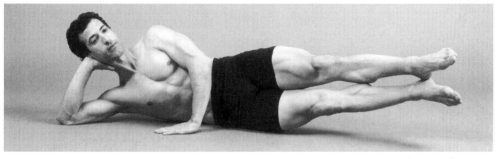

Photo 5.69

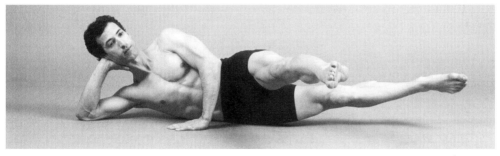

Photo 5.70

Perform the previous six exercises on the other side.

25. Forearm Side Pull-Ups and Forearm Side Plank

exhaling through the lips in the Pilates manner

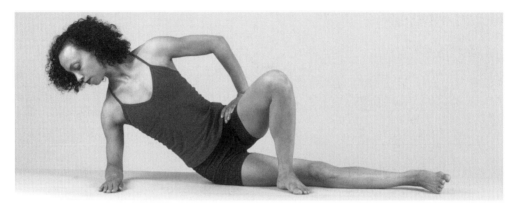

Photo 5.71

Forearm Side Pull-Ups and Forearm Side Plank strengthen the sides of your waist and hips, and tones the muscles in your arms. These exercises are for advanced practitioners who have already mastered Forearm Plank and the Side-Lying Series. They would be added to the end of the Side-Lying Series, or in place of it.

Scoot down to the lower half of your mat and lie on your right side with your legs in line with your torso. The bottom half of your legs should be off the mat. Lift up on your right forearm, with the elbow under your shoulder and forearm at a right angle to your torso. Place your left hand on your hip and cross your left leg over your right, knee to the ceiling and foot flat on the floor (photo 5.71). Press firmly into the floor with your forearm, hold the ribs in, and engage the muscles under your right arm to stabilize the shoulder.

Exhale as you lift up your torso and hips, dragging your right leg in along the floor (photo 5.72). Pull up and in with your abdominals, allowing your upper body to turn slightly toward the floor. Inhale as you lower your hips back down and reach the right leg out along the floor. Repeat Forearm Side Pull-Ups 2 more times.

On the last lift up, hold the position and place your left leg on top of the right balancing on the side of your right foot (photo 5.73). Hold Forearm Side Plank for 3 breath cycles. Finish by bending your knees and lowering your hips to the mat (photo 5.74). Repeat Forearm Side Pull-Ups and Forearm Side Plank on the other side.

☯ *For less difficulty, keep your left leg bent, foot flat on the floor instead of doing Forearm Side Plank.*

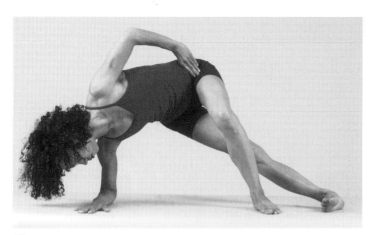

Photo 5.72

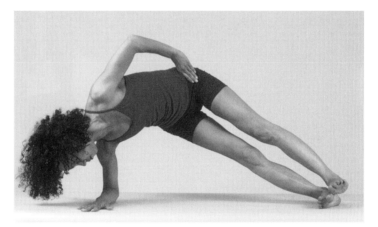

Photo 5.73

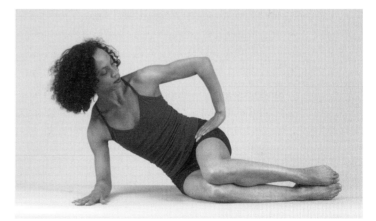

Photo 5.74

26. Mermaid and Pigeon Pose

Ujjayi breathing through the nose

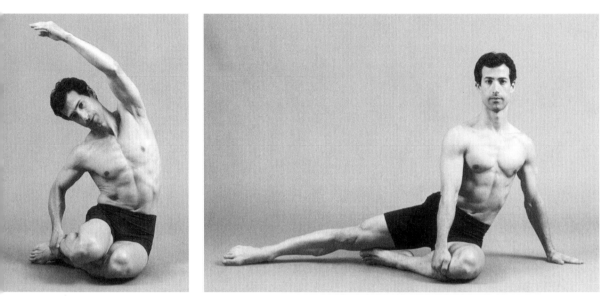

Photo 5.75

Photo 5.76

Mermaid stretches the sides of your torso and Pigeon Pose stretches the sides of your hips, buttocks, and lower back. Practice them individually at first before placing them together. They each go well after the Side-Lying Series or Forearm Side Pull-Ups.

Sit up on the side of your left hip and fold your legs under you. Hold on to your ankles with your right hand and inhale as you reach up with your left arm. Exhale as you curve your torso over to the right (photo 5.75). Feel the stretch in the left side of the torso and hip. Hold Mermaid for 2 breath cycles.

Next, place your left hand on the floor next to you and stretch your right leg straight out to your side (photo 5.76). Turn your hips and torso to the left and position your left shin on a diagonal line under you, and your right leg back in parallel. Exhale as you fold your body over your left leg (photos 5.77 and 5.78). Feel the stretch in your left hip and buttock as you relax and breathe in Pigeon Pose for 3 breath cycles. Lift up and repeat Mermaid and Pigeon Pose on the other side.

❂ *If having your shin under you in Pigeon Pose bothers your knee, sit on the side of your hip instead.*

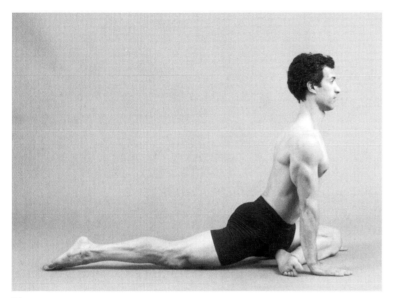

Photo 5.77

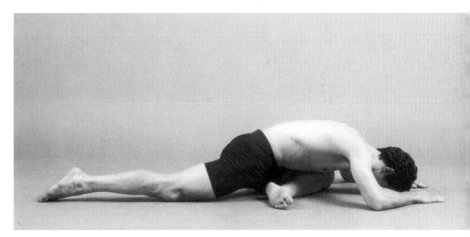

Photo 5.78

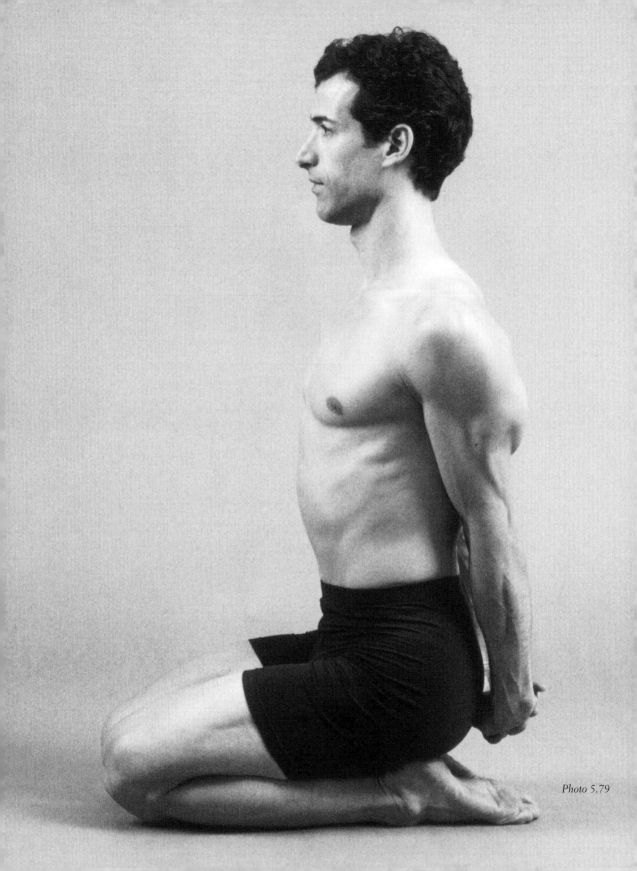

Photo 5.79

27. Yoga Mudra

Ujjayi breathing through the nose

Yoga Mudra stretches the chest, shoulders, and back. It goes well after Forearm Side Plank, but can really go anywhere in the floor routine as well as at the end of the workout.

Sit on your knees and lace your fingers behind your back (photo 5.79). Exhale as you round your spine over your knees and lift your arms up behind you (photo 5.80). Bring your forehead close to your knees and the top of your head to the floor. Hold for 2 to 4 breath cycles.

If sitting on your legs bothers your knees, place a pillow between your hips and back of your lower legs.

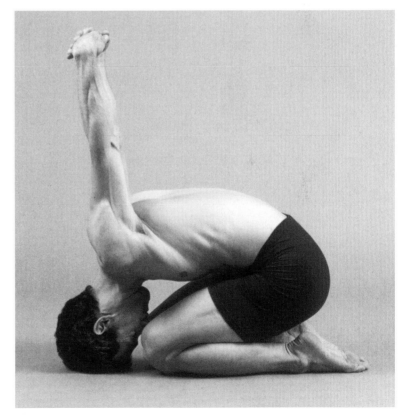

Photo 5.80

28. Cross-Gate Pose and Side Arm Balance

Ujjayi breathing through the nose

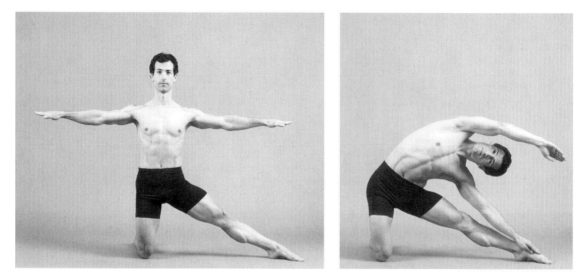

Photo 5.81

Photo 5.82

Cross-Gate Pose stretches the sides of your torso and hips, and Side Arm Balance strengthens the sides of your waist and your arms. They are placed well with the other kneeling exercises, such as Yoga Mudra, Cat Back, or Knee Balance.

From your knees, extend the left leg out to the side and turn it out so the toe points to the side. Inhale as you reach your arms out to the sides (photo 5.81). Exhale as you curve over to the left, tilting the hips somewhat (photo 5.82). Slide your left hand toward the foot and reach your right arm overhead as you hold Cross-Gate Pose for 2 breath cycles. Exhale and lift your torso back up.

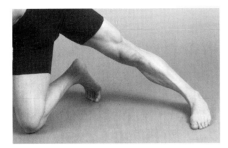

Photo 5.83

Lean over to the right and place your right hand on the mat and your left hand on your hip. Turn your left leg parallel and press your left foot flat on the floor (photo 5.83). Firm the muscles of your right arm and shoulder to stabilize your body, then exhale as you place your

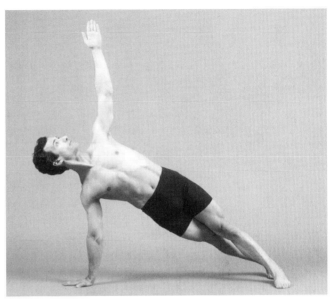

Photo 5.84

right foot behind the left, placing the outside of the ball of your right foot on the floor. Make sure your legs and hips are in line with your torso as you hold Side Arm Balance. When you are ready, reach up to the ceiling with the left arm and gaze up at your hand (photo 5.84). Hold this position for 3 breath cycles. Keep your belly hollowed, ribs in, and feel the entire right side of your body holding you up. Finish by bringing the right knee back to the mat and lifting your torso back up.

Change legs and repeat the above 2 exercises on the other side.

❷ *If you are not ready for Side Arm Balance, keep your knee on the floor and raise the extended leg in the air to hip height (photo 5.85). Hold Side Knee Balance pose for 3 breath cycles, and then repeat on the other side.*

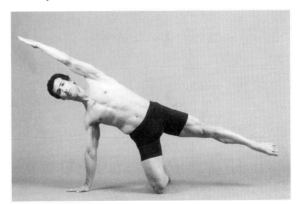

Photo 5.85

29. Camel and Rabbit Pose

Ujjayi breathing through the nose

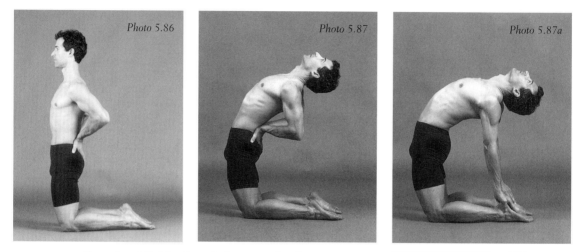

Photo 5.86

Photo 5.87

Photo 5.87a

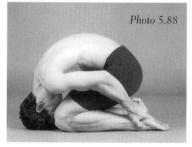

Photo 5.88

Camel and Rabbit Pose balance each other out, as do all extension and flexion exercises for the spine. They go well with the other kneeling exercises, like Cat Back, Knee Balance, and Cross-Gate Pose.

From standing on your knees, place your hands on the back of your hips, fingers pointing down (photo 5.86). Inhale as you arch your spine back from the top of your head while keeping your hips in line with your thighs (photo 5.87). Press firmly with your hands, and squeeze your buttocks to support the lower back. If possible, reach your hands down to your heels and brace your arms straight for support (photo 5.87A). Keep your hips pressed forward and avoid arching your neck too far back.

To come out of this pose, bring your head up first and then sit your hips, down on your heels. Next, hold on to your heels as you round your spine forward in Rabbit Pose. Pull in with your abdominals and get your forehead as close to your knees as possible (photo 5.88), as you place the top of your head on the floor. Lift your hips up, rolling forward on the top of your head, keeping a firm hold on your heels. Feel this stretch in your upper back and sholders. Sit your hips back down and roll your back up to sitting.

30. Crouch with Toe Raises
normal diaphragmatic breathing through the nose

Crouch with Toe Raises is an excellent exercise to strengthen your arches and stretch your feet. It goes best right before standing up from your floor routine as it loosens and prepares the feet for supporting your weight.

Start with your feet parallel and a few inches apart. Sit in a crouch position on the balls of your feet, with your fingers touching the floor for support and balance (photo 5.89). Relax in this position, with your back rounded and your chest close to your thighs, and feel the stretch in the back of your lower legs.

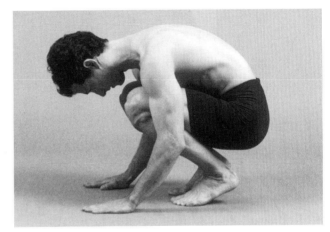

Photo 5.89

Inhale as you lift up onto your toes as high as you can, keeping your hands touching the ground for support and balance (photo 5.90). Be careful not to let your ankles roll out as you lift up. Exhale as you relax the heels back down, but not all the way to the floor. Repeat lifting up on your toes from Crouch 10 times.

☯ *If this position hurts your knees, stand all the way up and press just one foot to the ball of the foot, lifting the arch high and bending the toes. Stretch up onto both toes, then change feet, like doing a slow prance step. Alternate single foot arch lifts 10 times with each foot.*

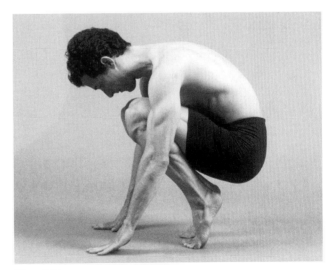

Photo 5.90

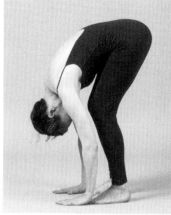

Photo 5.91

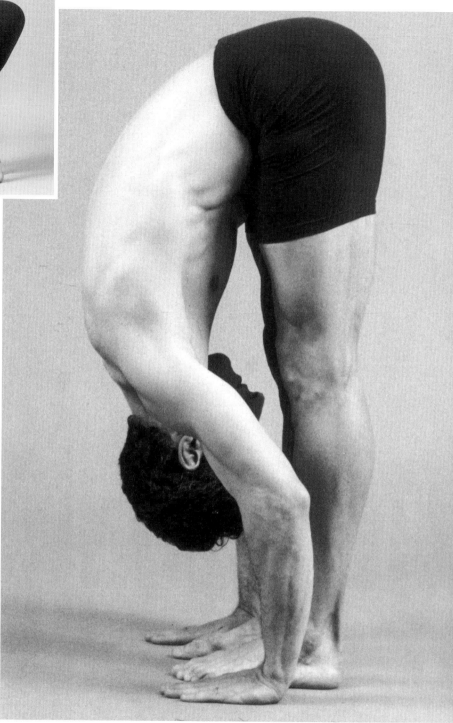

Photo 5.92

31. Forward Bend and Flat Back

Ujjayi breathing through the nose

Forward Bend and Flat Back are great stretches for the back of your legs and also stretch and strengthen your lower back. They go well after Rag Doll and before or after Sun Salutation.

Stand and hang forward over bent legs in Rag Doll position (photo 5.91). Touch the floor in front of your feet with your hands and exhale deeply as you straighten your legs. Use your core muscles to bring your torso in close to your legs, and be careful not to sit back on your heels (photo 5.92).

Next, inhale and reach your back flat and slightly away from your torso, but keep your fingers touching the mat (photo 5.93). Exhale and release back over your legs in a full forward bend. Repeat Forward Bend and Flat Back one more time.

Finish by exhaling as you roll up sequentially from Forward Bend to standing. Engage the abdominals and buttocks as you do this and let the arms and the head hang as you come up through the spine (photo 5.94).

❷ *If your hands don't reach the floor, place your hands on yoga blocks or a low chair for support. If your knees hyperextend easily, keep your knees slightly bent all the time.*

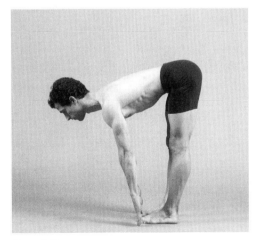
Photo 5.93

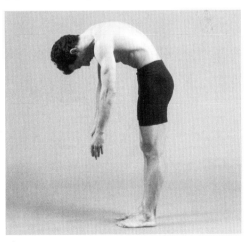
Photo 5.94

32. Sun Salutation

Ujjayi breathing through the nose

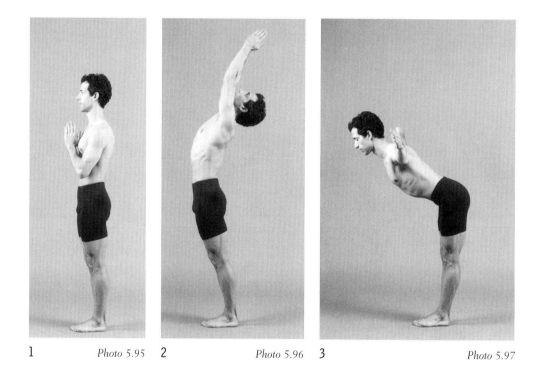

1   *Photo 5.95*   **2**   *Photo 5.96*   **3**   *Photo 5.97*

This is a classic version of the hatha yoga Salute to the Sun, with an extra stretch in the lunge section. This exercise is supposed to flow with your breath as it develops strength and flexibility for the whole body. In Yogilates, your Sun Salutation comes after the floor work and also after Small Knee Bends and Toe Raises.

1. Stand toward the front of your mat with your feet together in Tadasana pose (photo 5.95). 2. Inhale as you reach your arms up and back, squeezing your buttocks to protect your lower back (photo 5.96).

3. and 4. Exhale as you open your arms out and gracefully dive over your legs in a forward bend, placing your hands on the floor on either side of your feet (photos 5.97 and 5.98).

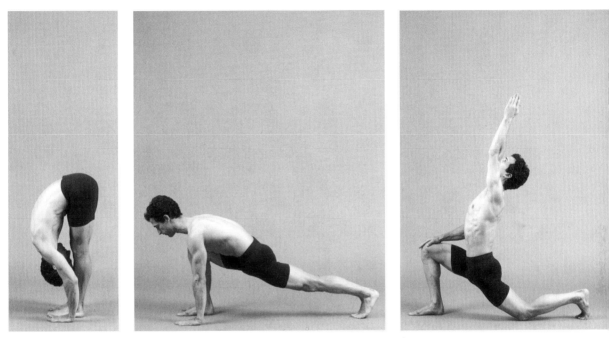

4   *Photo 5.98*   5   *Photo 5.99*   6   *Photo 5.100*

5. Inhale as you reach back with your left leg onto the ball of the foot in a deep lunge position (photo 5.99). Be sure to keep your right foot flat on the mat, knee over the ankle.

6. Exhale as you gently set the left knee down on the mat, and place your right hand on the right knee for support. Inhale as you lift your left arm up and back, pressing forward with the front of your hips. You should feel a stretch in the front of your torso and left hip (photo 5.100).

❷ *The forward bends can be made easier by allowing your knees to bend, which you need to do if your hands don't reach the floor. In the lunge position, keep your hands on your hips instead of reaching up.*

❷ *In moving from the Plank position to Chaturanga, you can set your knees on the floor before lowering your torso. Work slowly and stay in touch with your breath, and remember that you can always do the Modified Sun Salute action from Chapter 4 if this sequence is too hard.*

159

7. Exhale as you place both hands back on the mat and step back with the right leg into a push-up position with your feet hip-distance apart. This is called Plank (photo 5.101). Inhale and pause in this position. 8. Exhale as you bend your elbows straight back and lower your body so that your chest is one inch above the mat. This is called Chaturanga (photo 5.102). Keep your body in one piece and your shoulders drawn down the back.

9. Supporting yourself with your arms, inhale as you pull yourself forward into Upward-Facing Dog; rolling onto the top of your feet, pressing the chest forward, and squeezing your buttocks to protect your lower back (photo 5.103). Be sure to keep your shoulders down as you press your arms straight. 10. Curl your toes under and exhale as you push your hips back and up into Downward-Facing Dog (photo 5.104). Hold this position for 4 to 5 breath cycles.

11. Inhale as you step forward with the left foot between your hands into a lunge posi-

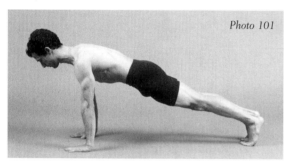

Photo 101

7

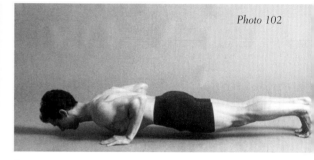

Photo 102

8

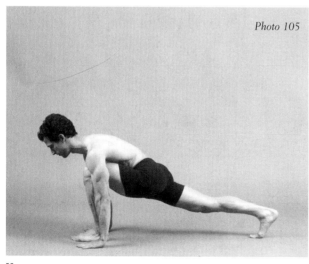

Photo 105

11

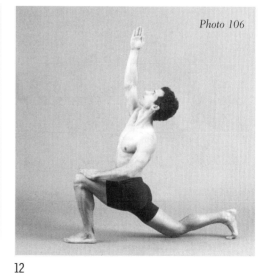

Photo 106

12

tion, knee over the ankle (photo 5.105). **12.** Exhale to gently set the right knee down, and place the left hand on your left thigh. Inhale and lift the right arm up and back, feeling a stretch in the front of the torso and right hip (photo 5.106). **13.** Exhale and place both hands back on the mat as you step your right foot next to the left and stretch over in a forward bend (photo 5.107).

14. Let your knees bend and inhale as you reach your back flat and your arms out (photo 5.108), **15.** lifting yourself up to standing with the arms overhead (photo 5.109). **16.** Exhale and bring the hands in front of your chest (photo 5.110).

Repeat Sun Salutation, this time stepping back and forward with the other leg. As you become more experienced, you can practice one more round of Sun Salutation.

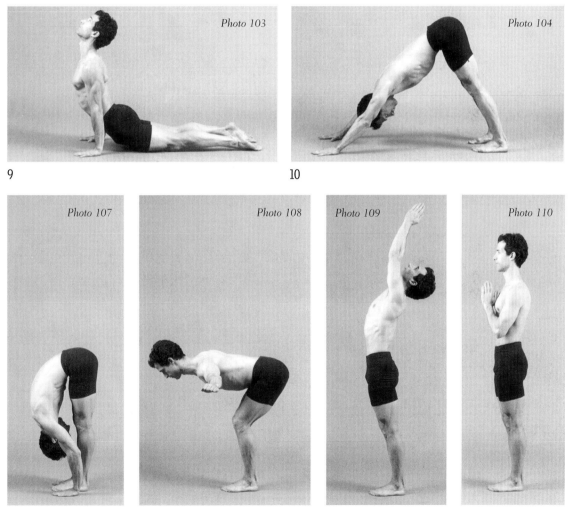

Photo 103

9

Photo 104

10

Photo 107

13

Photo 108

14

Photo 109

15

Photo 110

16

33. Pliés to Goddess

Ujjayi breathing through the nose

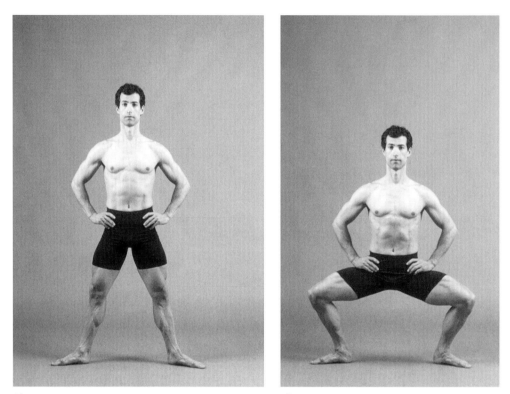

Photo 5.111   *Photo 5.112*

Pliés to Goddess strengthens and tones your inner thighs, buttocks, calves, and feet and also develops your balance. It works well if placed after Chair Pose and Warrior One and before Warrior Two in the standing part of your routine.

Face sideways and stand in the middle of your mat with your feet about 3 to 4 feet apart* in parallel. Place your hands on your hips, lift up on your toes and rotate your heels under you so your legs are turned out (photo 5.111). Settle your heels into the floor and inhale as you bend your knees into a plié (photo 5.112). Exhale as you push your legs back straight. Repeat 8 slow pliés. Keep your back and pelvis straight up and down, and feel the connection between your feet to engage your inner thighs.

*Your feet shouldn't be as wide apart for other exercises.

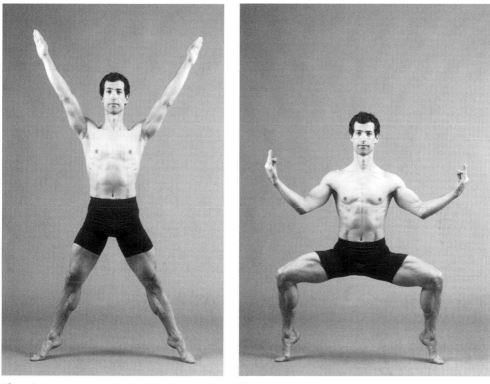

Photo 5.113   Photo 5.114

Then, keep your legs straight as you inhale and lift up on to the balls of your feet and reach your arms up in V position (photo 5.113). Exhale as you bend your knees into plié, but stay up on your toes. Bend your elbows and touch the first finger and thumb of each hand. Hold this Goddess position for 3 to 5 breath cycles (photo 5.114). Finish by lowering the heels, straightening your legs, and rotating them back into parallel.

❷ *If you feel stress in your knees, you may want to place your feet a little closer together and don't do pliés as deeply. You may also keep your hands on your hips to help your balance.*

34. Standing Bow, Wide Forward Bend, and Wide Flat Back

Ujjayi breathing through the nose

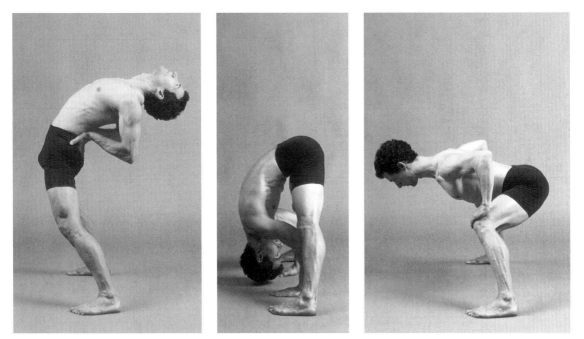

Photo 5.115

Photo 5.116

Photo 5.117

This sequence starts with a stretch for the front of your torso and hips, and then stretches and strengthens your back and hamstrings.

Face sideways and stand in the middle of your mat in wide parallel stance with your feet 3 to 5 feet apart, appropriate to your height (see box on page 96). Place your hands on the back of your hips and inhale as you arch your head and spine backward. Press firmly on your hips and squeeze your buttocks to protect your back (photo 5.115). Exhale as you bring your torso back up and then bend forward over your legs. Place your hands on the floor (photo 5.116) and relax in this position for 3 breath cycles. Allow the torso to hang out of the hips with your legs straight. Make sure you don't lock your knees or lift your heels off the floor.

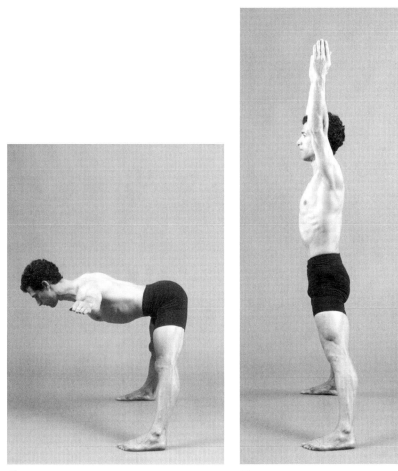

Photo 5.118   Photo 5.119

Then, place your hands on your thighs, and inhale as you bend your knees and reach your back out parallel to the floor (photo 5.117). Keep your legs bent as you hold your back flat for 3 full breaths in this position. Then, exhale and push your legs straight as you reach your arms out to your sides (photo 5.118). Draw your ribs and belly in and keep your shoulders down as you hold this position for 2 more breath cycles.

To finish, inhale as you bring your torso to standing up straight and reach your arms over your head (photo 5.119).

☯ *Modify the straight-leg positions by bending the knees. For less difficulty, when you lift up in the end, place your hands on your hips rather than reaching them out and up.*

35. Side Lunges and Yoga Hop

Ujjayi breathing through the nose

Side Lunges and Yoga Hop strengthen the sides of your legs and buttocks and develop spring in the ankles and feet. They may be placed anywhere in the standing part of your routine.

Face sideways and stand in the middle of your mat with your feet together and place your hands on your hips (photo 5.120). Step the right leg out to the side in a parallel lunge (photo 5.121). Keep your left leg straight and land the right foot softly as you bend your right knee.

Exhale as you push off with the right foot to bring your feet back together. Repeat 8 Side Lunges on the right side, keeping both feet parallel. Then repeat 8 side lunges to the left, finishing with the legs together.

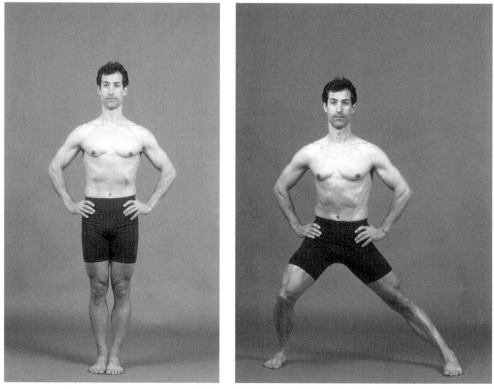

Photo 5.120 *Photo 5.121*

Next, stand with your feet together in the middle of your mat and your hands on the sides of your hips. Bend your knees, pressing your feet flat into the floor. Inhale as you jump up with the legs together in the air (photo 5.122). Then, open the legs wide and exhale as you land quietly with the knees bent (photo 5.123). Repeat Yoga Hop back from this wide stance position, jumping up and landing with the feet back together. Be mindful to land softly through your feet, landing toe, ball, and heel to protect the knees, and to spring up from the feet when you jump.

Use Yoga Hop in place of stepping whenever you transition to a wide parallel stance.

❂ *If your feet or knees are delicate, you can make the lunges and hops smaller.*

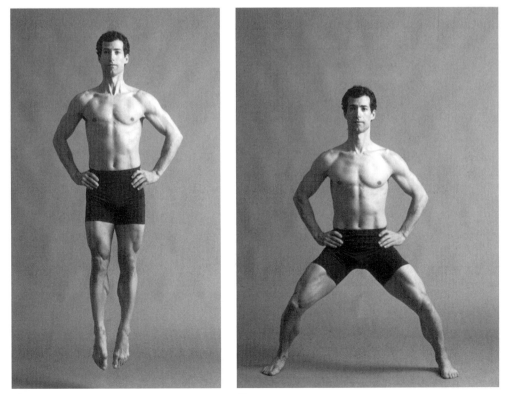

Photo 5.122   Photo 5.123

36. Warrior Two, Lay Back, and Triangle
Ujjayi breathing through the nose

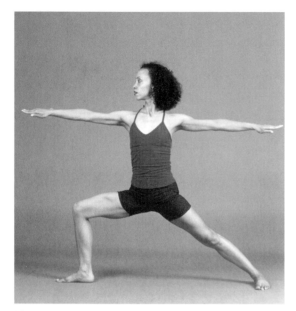

Photo 5.124

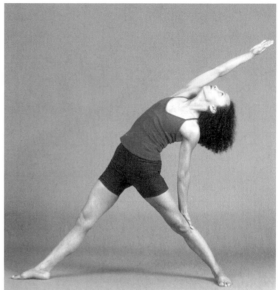

Photo 5.125

These exercises strengthen and tone all the leg muscles, stretch the torso, and stretch the torso and inner thighs as well. They may be placed in the middle of your standing exercises, after Warrior One and Pliés. See the previous chapter for more detailed descriptions of Warrior Two and Triangle.

Stand in the middle of your mat with your feet in parallel wide stance and your hands on your hips. Rotate the right leg 90 degrees out to the right, and rotate the left foot in 20 degrees, making sure your hips stay level and square to the front. Exhale as you bend your right knee in line with your right foot, and reach your arms out to the sides. Look to your right and hold Warrior Two for 4 to 5 breath cycles (photo 5.124).

Next, straighten your right leg and inhale as you arch back with your torso, lifting the right arm up and placing the left hand on the back of your left leg (photo 5.125). Do not press down with your left hand on your leg, but instead reach up through the torso and the spine. Exhale as you bring the torso back to straight up.

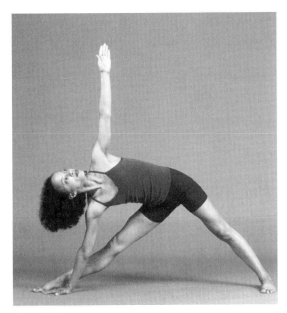

Photo 5.126

Inhale as you shift your pelvis to the left, and tilt over sideways into Triangle Pose (photo 5.126). Keep your back straight and your pelvis neutral and flat to the front. Place your right hand on your shin, or, if you can do so without compromising your alignment, touch the floor next to your foot with your fingers. Reach your left arm to the ceiling and turn your face to look up. Ground yourself without locking your knees, as you hold Triangle for 3 to 5 breath cycles. Finish by exhaling as you bring your torso back to standing straight up with your arms out to the sides. Turn your legs parallel in a wide stance, and then step or Yoga Hop the legs together. Step or Yoga Hop your legs back out to wide stance and repeat the same sequence of Warrior Two, Lay Back, and Triangle on the left side.

☯ *For less difficulty, modify these exercises by leaving your hands on your hips the whole time.*

37. Long Angle

Ujjayi breathing through the nose

Long Angle stretches the inner thighs and groin and strengthens the legs and buttocks. It can join or replace Triangle, after Warrior Two and Lay Back, in your standing routine.

Facing sideways, stand in the middle of your mat with your feet in parallel wide stance and your hands on your hips. Rotate the right leg 90 degrees out to the right, and rotate the left foot in 20 degrees. Exhale as you bend your right knee in line with your right foot and tilt the pelvis and torso to the right. Place your elbow on your right thigh and bring your torso and hips in line with the left leg (photo 5.127).

Keep your pelvis square to the front as you reach your left arm straight overhead, being careful not to hunch up your shoulders. If it doesn't compromise your knee or pelvic alignment, you can reach your right hand to the floor next to your foot (photo 5.128); otherwise, leave your right elbow on your thigh for support. Feel grounded, holding power in your core as you hold Long Angle pose for 3 to 5 breath cycles. Finish by exhaling as you lift your torso back up and bring yourself to parallel wide stance. Repeat Long Angle to left side.

☞ *Modify Long Angle by placing your elbow on your thigh for support and leaving your other arm by your side (photo 5.127).*

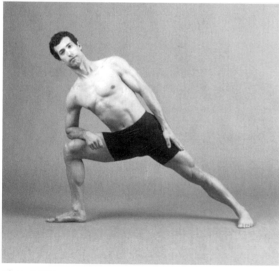

Photo 5.127

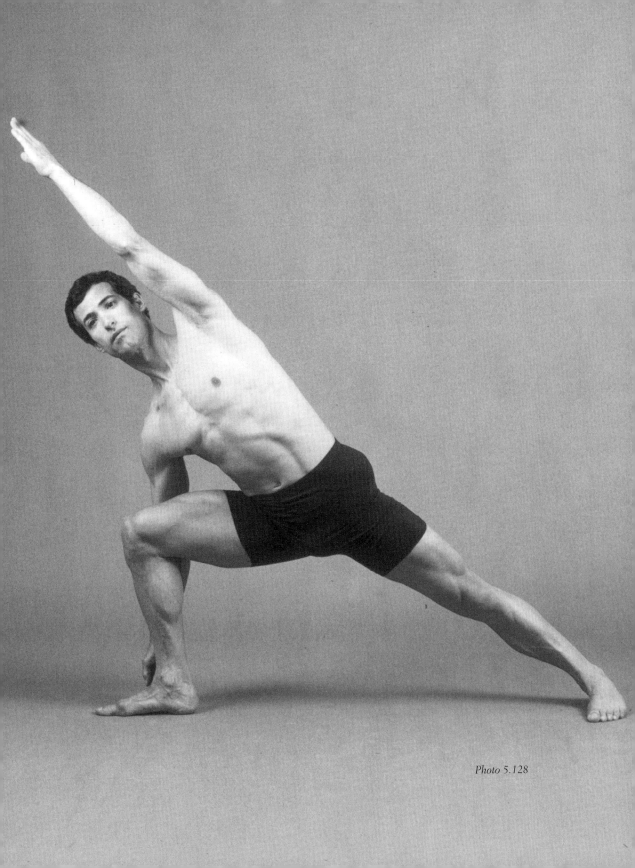

Photo 5.128

38. Bound Long Angle into Standing Side Leg Extension

Ujjayi breathing through the nose

This advanced move is for experts only and works flexibility in the hips and legs as well as balance. It would be placed after Long Angle.

From Long Angle on the right side (see last exercise), wrap your right arm in front and under the right leg, and your left arm behind your back. Clasp your hands behind your right hip (photo 5.129). Stay relaxed and breathe deeply as you hold this Bound Long Angle pose for 3 to 5 breath cycles.

Then, keeping the hands clasped, walk your left foot in toward your right, bringing both feet underneath you to hip-distance apart (photo 5.130). Shift your weight to your

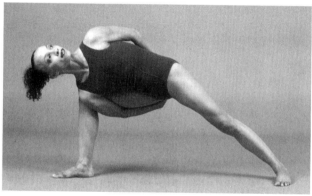

Photo 5.129

left foot and carefully stand up on one leg, holding the right leg in a soft position with your arms. Take your time and be ready to unclasp your hands if you lose your balance. When you are standing straight up and balanced, exhale as you extend the right leg straight with the foot flexed (photo 5.131). Hold this pose for 3 to 5 breath cycles. Finish by releasing the leg and bringing it down next to your left. Repeat Bound Long Angle and Side Leg Extension to the other side.

☯ *Do not try this exercise if Long Angle with your arms clasped is at all difficult. If you feel a strain in your back while trying to stand up, skip that part of the exercise.*

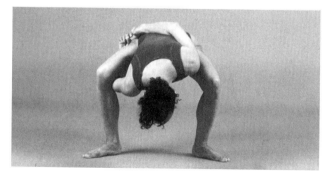

Photo 5.130

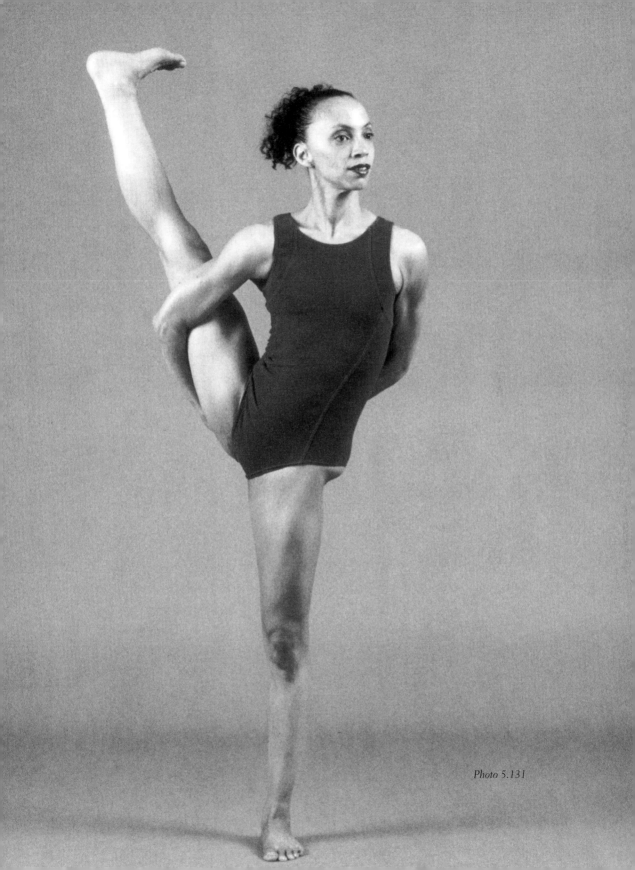

Photo 5.131

39. Parallel Tree, Warrior Three, and Half Moon
Ujjayi breathing through the nose

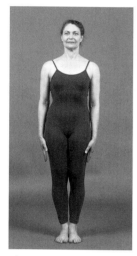

Photo 5.132

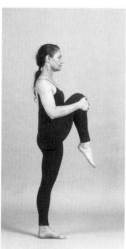

Photo 5.133

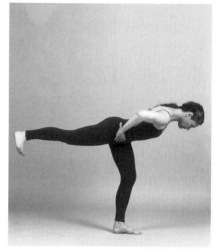

Photo 5.134

These three exercises develop your balance skills and improve the muscular endurance in your legs. Practice each of these exercises individually for a few sessions before trying to put them together. They can go before or after the other Warrior exercises and could replace Tree as a leg balance exercise in your routine.

Stand at the front of your mat in Tadasana (photo 5.132). Lift your right knee up and exhale as you hug it into your chest (photo 5.133). Inhale as you release hold of your right knee and position the leg in a parallel knee lift with your foot next to your left knee. Place your hands on your hips and balance in Parallel Tree for 3 breath cycles.

From Parallel Tree, allow your standing leg to bend a little, and exhale as you hinge forward 90 degrees from the hips with a flat back. Extend your right leg straight back in line with your torso and square your face, chest, and hips to the floor (photo 5.134). Once you feel steady, inhale as you reach your arms out to the sides and straighten your standing leg (photo 5.135). Ground yourself, pulling your abdominals in and feeling length all the way from the top of your head down through your right leg. Hold this Warrior Three position for 3 to 5 breath cycles.

Next, tilt forward and place your left hand on the mat as you rotate your body open to

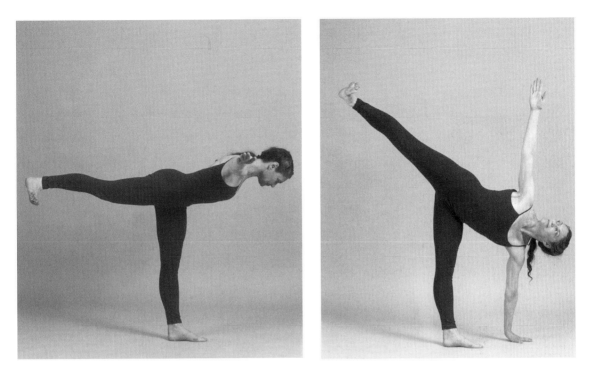

Photo 5.135

Photo 5.136

the right side. Keep your back straight and your right leg in line with your torso. Reach your right hand to the ceiling and hold this Half Moon position for 3 to 5 breath cycles (photo 5.136). To finish, rotate your body back to the front, and then bend your left knee as you lower the right leg and place your foot on the mat behind you in a lunge position. From there, step your feet together and stand up. Repeat Parallel Tree, Warrior Three, and Half Moon on the other side.

❷ *For less difficulty, in War-*
rior Three, keep your
hands on your hips. In
Half Moon, place a block
about 12 inches in front
of your standing foot and
place your hand on it for
easier balance (photos
5.137 and 5.138).

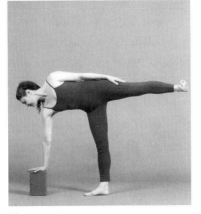

Photo 5.137

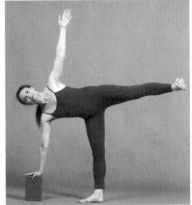

Photo 5.138

40. Pilates Stance and Standing Leg Lift

exhaling through the lips in the Pilates manner

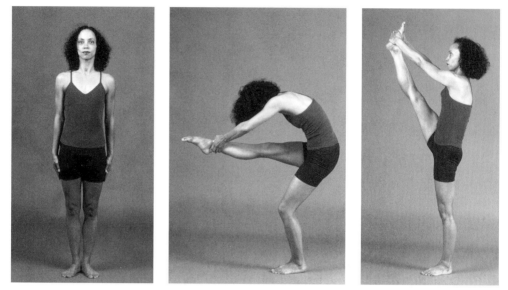

Photo 5.139   Photo 5.140   Photo 5.141

Pilates Stance brings your legs into a more powerful standing position, and Standing Leg Lift develops balance and stretches your legs. These exercises would come toward the end of your standing routine and could be used as a replacement for Tree as a balance exercise.

Stand near the front of your mat with the feet together in Tadasana. Keep your heels touching and separate your toes 2 to 3 inches apart. Rotate your thighs out to bring your sit bones under your pelvis and your inner thighs together. This is called Pilates Stance (photo 5.139).

Exhale as you curve over with your torso and lift your right leg off the floor. Allow your left knee to bend as you do this (photo 5.140). Grasp your right ankle and inhale as you straighten your body back up, lifting the right leg up with you (photo 5.141). Keep your shoulders down, elbows out to the side, and stomach pulled in. Straighten both your legs, while making sure your pelvis stays in neutral. Balance in Standing Leg Lift position for 3 to 5 breath cycles. To finish, release the right leg and slowly lower it next to the left in Pilates Stance. Repeat Pilates Stance and Standing Leg Lift with the left leg.

☯ *For less difficulty, modify this exercise by holding the right leg*
   under the thigh and keeping it bent as you balance.

176

41. Squat Pose

Ujjayi breathing through the nose

Squat Pose stretches the back, groin, and calves. It can go anywhere in your standing routine.

Stand with your feet slightly wider than your hips and turn your feet slightly out. Squat down between your feet and rest your elbows inside your knees (photo 5.142). Your feet should be flat and you should relax in the position. Hold Squat Pose for 4 to 5 breath cycles. You may finish this exercise by standing back up or sitting down on your mat.

☯ *If you have difficulty getting your feet flat on the floor,*
  you can widen your stance and not sit the hips so far down.

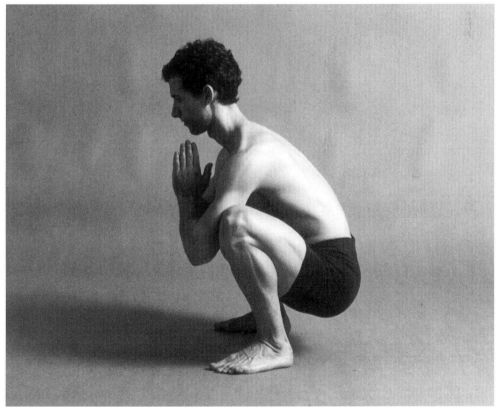

Photo 5.142

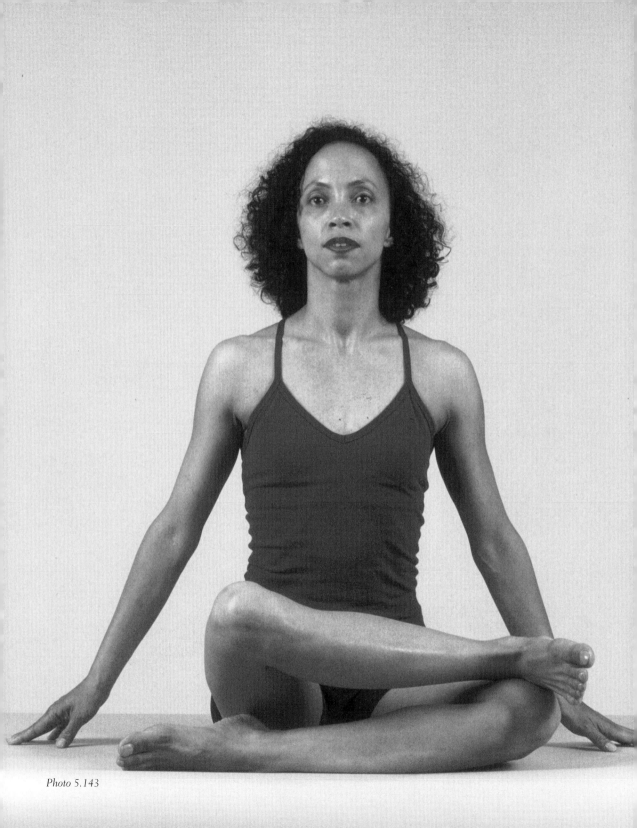

Photo 5.143

42. Seated Hip Stretch

normal diaphragmatic breathing through the nose

Seated Hip Stretch is an intense stretch for your outer hips and buttocks. It may be sub-stituted for Pigeon Pose or added to Seated Spiral in your floor routine.

Sit on your mat with your legs crossed in Easy Pose. Then, cross your right leg over your left leg, placing the ankle near your left knee, and align your shins parallel to each other (photo 5.143). Exhale as you round forward over your legs (photo 5.144). Feel the intense stretch in your right hip and buttock. Relax and hold Seated Hip Stretch for at least 4 to 5 breath cycles.

Repeat this exercise crossing the left leg over.

☯ *For less difficulty, sit on a folded blanket or firm pillow and allow the knee of the leg crossed over to tilt up.*

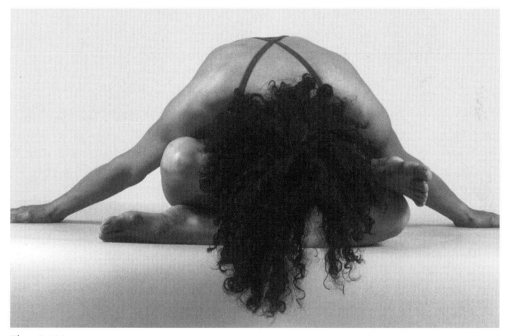

Photo 5.144

43. Full Shoulder Stand and Plow

normal diaphragmatic breathing through the nose

Full Shoulder Stand allows for reverse circulation in your body, and Plow stretches your lower back. Do these at the end of your routine to help your body recover and relax.

Lie on your back and lift your hips in the air in a Half Shoulder Stand with your hips supported on your hands and your knees bent. Exhale as you extend your legs straight up without tensing your legs or feet. Walk your hands up from your hips to your lower back, bringing your legs, hips, and torso in a more vertical line (photo 5.145). Make sure you are balanced and comfortable without putting a strain on your neck. Hold Shoulder Stand for 4 to 5 breath cycles.

Next, lower your hips back into your hands and exhale as you bend your knees in toward your shoulders. Gently

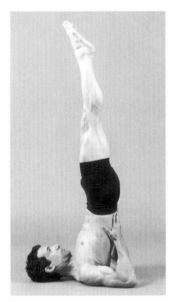

Photo 5.145

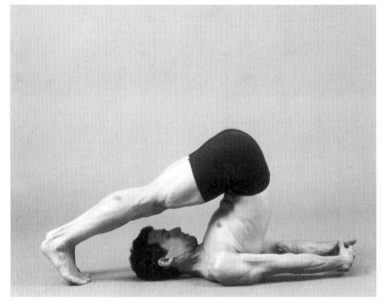

Photo 5.146

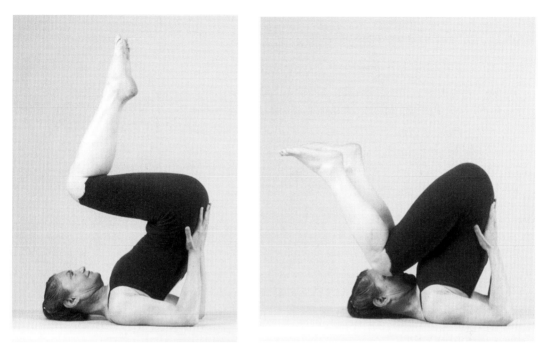

Photo 5.147   Photo 5.148

extend your legs over your head, bringing the feet toward the mat as in Easy Plow. If your feet can comfortably rest on the mat over your head, you may reach the arms down and clasp the hands behind the back (photo 5.146). Relax in Plow pose for 4 to 5 breath cycles. Finish by bringing your hands back to your hips, bend your knees, and slowly roll down onto your back.

☯ *For less difficulty, modify Shoulder Stand by keeping the hips in the hands and the knees bent (photo 5.147). Modify Plow by keeping the hands in the hips and knees bent and bending the knees to the shoulders (photo 5.148).*

Resting and Meditation

No matter how advanced your workout gets, always finish your practice with Shavasana (Corpse Pose, photo 5.149) and Meditation (photo 5.150).

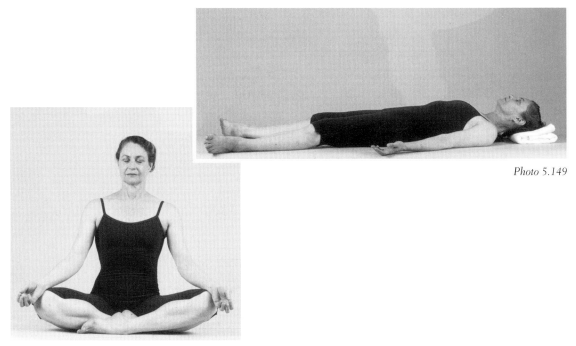

Photo 5.149

Photo 5.150

There are hundreds of different hatha yoga and Pilates mat exercises you can choose from in designing your Yogilates routine. But, you have more than enough here to get started and to take your fitness to a whole new level. For additional needs, a certified Yogilates instructor can help you with routines especially designed for different purposes, whether you are recovering from injury or want a complimentary regimen for a specific sport. In general, the key to advancing your practice is repetition, repetition, repetition. Be patient and consistent, restraining the urge to always do more. Attention to your form and efficiency in your movements will inevitably lead you to healthy and permanent changes in your mind and body.

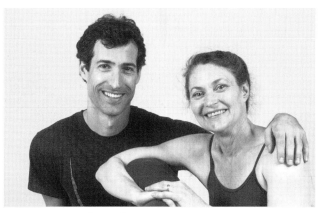

Jonathan with yoga instructor Patricia Levy

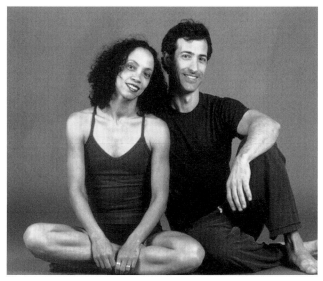

Jonathan with Pilates instructor Judy Tyrus

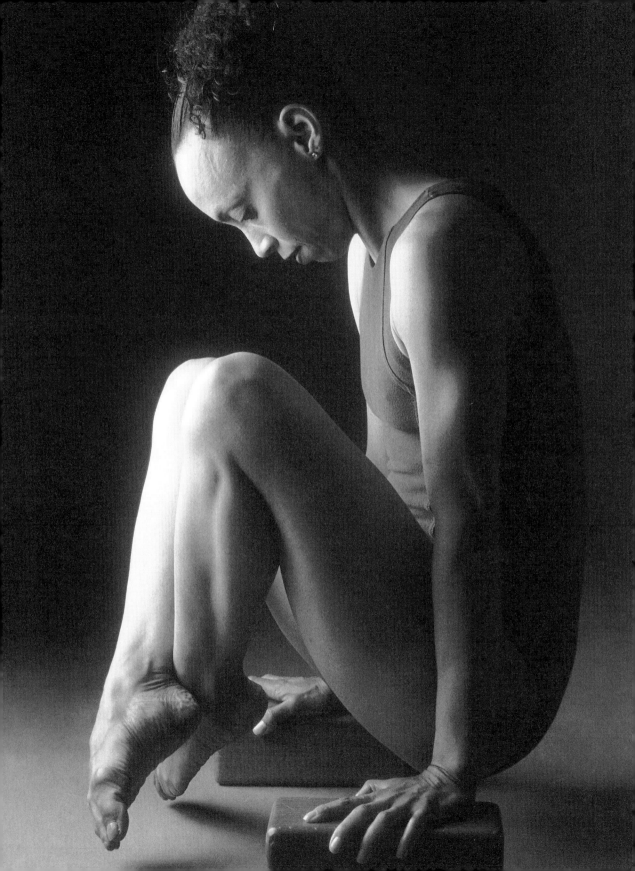

Chapter Six

Completing Your Yogilates Fitness Program

Moving my body rhythmically and repetitively helps me tap into my intuition, and more of my mind becomes available to me.
—Christiane Northrup, M.D.

As great as yoga and Pilates are for your health, they still do not cover all the elements necessary to complete your fitness program. For optimal long-term health, aerobic conditioning should be a part of your Yogilates program. Although some will claim that it is possible to do hatha yoga or a Pilates workout at such a speed as to make it aerobic, that kind of effort is wrongheaded. Yoga and Pilates yield best results when performed at a mindful pace, which also helps ensure safety and quality in your practice. Reaching for a real cardiovascular workout from your practice is just asking too much of these systems. Far easier (and healthier) than pushing up the speed of your Yogilates workout is to simply add regular aerobic exercise into your fitness lifestyle. The benefits from doing this are numerous, including a healthier heart, better circulation, lower cholesterol, less unwanted fat, a way to rid the body of toxins, improved skin tone and appearance, and more relief from physical and emotional stress.

Aerobic conditioning can also promote personal fulfillment in different ways. Cardiovascular fitness is fundamentally about developing your stamina. This is another innate capacity you have that brings both inner and outer strength. You will find that the continuity and flow to moderate aerobic activity develops a unique synchronicity between mind and body that isn't possible through other forms of exercise. This active state of consciousness can be described as "moving meditation" and allows the brain to focus in a different, perhaps deeper, way on unresolved issues. Problem solving and realizations during aerobic activity are quite common, and are another benefit you can look forward to. In any case, your spiritual health can be positively affected by your aerobic training almost as much as from your meditation practice. Be confident in the knowledge that your body is being refined for both grace and endurance. Yogilates and aerobic conditioning is a healthy lifestyle that does cover all the bases and brings completeness to your fitness program.

The other good news is that the practice of Yogilates perfectly primes the body for aerobic activity. Through your practice you will have developed better breathing capacity, more strength, better balance, and more efficient alignment, all of which make aerobic activity easier to do. You only need to understand some basic principles of cardiovascular training before you begin.

Aerobic Exercise

The general definition for aerobic exercise is straightforward and easy to follow: It should be a continuous activity that involves large muscle groups and brings your heart rate into a steady state. This steady state should be somewhere between 65 percent and 85 percent of your maximum heart rate (MHR). To find out what your MHR is, take your age and subtract it from 220. For example, if you are 55 years old, your MHR is 165. This number represents an estimate of the maximum beats per minute (bpm) your heart could attain if it was pushed to its limit. The range of 65 percent to 85 percent of this MHR is your training range (TR) and represents the range of bpm that allow you to remain in an aerobic state for optimal cardiovascular benefit. So, for a 55-year-old, the TR would be 108 to 140 bpm. What these figures give you is an indication of the intensity of your workout. Remember that, as we learned in Yogilates, more is not better. In fact, it is very important that you start on the lower end of your training range and very gradually work to the middle. This will allow for greater safety and comfort and still give you all the benefits you need from aerobic conditioning.

For those who have little experience in aerobic conditioning, using a heart rate monitor to manage your intensity is like having a mirror for the inside of your body. It gives you precision in knowing how hard your heart is working. Eventually, however, you want to get most of your information from how your body feels. One of the best alternative ways to gauge the intensity of your aerobic workout is to be aware of how you're breathing. If you can comfortably breathe through your nose while working out, then you're not likely to go above your TR. So, just as in your Yogilates practice, use your awareness of your breath to guide your aerobic exercise.

How do I decide which method of aerobic exercise is best for me?

The answer for this is simple: Pick what's fun! Remember, any activity that is continuous and uses large muscle groups can be aerobic. When children are happy, they like to run around, climb things, play in water, ride bikes, and dance. They also like to share these experiences with others. The adult equivalents of these would be jogging or walking briskly, hiking, swimming, bicycling, and dancing. All of these are pleasurable forms of aerobic conditioning, and many can be done in pairs or groups for added enjoyment. Of course, you will still have to stay in your training range and listen to your body. I also strongly recommend getting permission from your physician before beginning your exercise program. Your doctor may also have appropriate suggestions for which type of aerobic exercise is best for you.

How often and for how long should I do aerobic conditioning?

You should do aerobic conditioning 3 to 5 times a week. The minimum number is important because to see positive results in your cardiovascular fitness, a consistent schedule is required. But there is also a maximum limit to the frequency of your workouts because, like Yogilates, too much aerobic conditioning puts stress on your system. There is actually no improvement in cardiovascular fitness from doing more than 5 days a week, while the risk of injury rises rapidly.

In terms of duration, the minimum recommended is 20 minutes. As with frequency, there is also an upper limit to duration that prevails on reason and common sense. The upper limit varies according to the method of exercise and the intensity of training. For example, I have a client who recently added walking to her fitness program. She happens to love walking, and had a friend to walk with to keep her motivated. Although I would not recommend it, she and her friend started their aerobic conditioning by walking for 1 hour in the park. Her calves were tight the first couple of weeks, but she quickly adapted and now walks 3 times a week for at least 1 hour each time. Because walking is a low-intensity method of exercise, a relatively longer duration is within reason, although I would still recommend gradually building up to the hour length. On the other hand, swimming and jogging are methods of aerobic conditioning with much higher degrees of intensity than walking. For these, a recommended program would involve intervals of 3 to 5 minutes, with lower-intensity activity in between. As long as the total of the intervals equals at least 20 minutes, you will still get the same benefit as if you did one continuous set.

How do I know if I'm doing it right?

Aerobic exercise is more of a feel sport than a technical sport. If you are exercising in your training range and having fun, than all you have to do is be aware of how your body feels. Everyone moves a little differently and it isn't important that you look like others when you train. What does matter is how the movement feels to you. Does the movement feel smooth and controlled, or does it feel jerky and awkward? Are you loose and relaxed in your back, neck, and shoulders, or are you tense in these areas? Your Yogilates practice will have primed you for greater awareness of these things, and there is no reason to compromise posture or grace during your aerobic conditioning. What you should be striving for is economy of motion. Try to generate your movement from as close to the center of your body as you can. Remember that the arms and the legs can be moved from inside the torso. This means that the upper thighs and shoulders can usually be more relaxed. Most aerobic activities involve a counterbalancing of opposite arm to leg, as in walking or swimming. Rather than overswinging with your arms or your legs, try to feel the connection between the two appendages as a diagonal line that crosses at your center. You want to feel grounded and stable as you generate power from your core. Still draw the navel back, breath with your diaphragm, maintain the pelvis in neutral, and release the surface muscles to allow the deeper core muscles to take over. This will save energy and create strength at the same time.

Conclusion

Lifestyle changes are the key to long-term health and fitness. The only way to begin is one step at a time. Even if it is only a little one, it is one less step that you have to take later on. With aerobic conditioning, as with your Yogilates practice, you should strive to be consistent, efficient, and moderate. When your heart, your breath, and your desire are all highly active and you are moving in a fluid, efficient manner, there is a wonderful sense of letting go that occurs.

As you pursue your fitness goals, give in to the flow of energy whenever you can. You might notice other things, such as the beauty of nature, a sense of freedom, a connection to the earth, a hidden power from within. You cannot stop the vital forces that are all around you. But by changing how you move, how you breathe, and how you think, you can alter their flow. The ability to change your life is up to you. Take all the qualities of your practice, and apply them to your everyday living. You can learn to be more faithful, more trusting, more tolerant, and more moderate toward yourself and others. In the universe, all actions create reactions. Therefore, your changes invariably affect changes in others. Let your own inner light also be a light for others. For the more you let it shine through, the more the whole universe will shine back.

Om Shanti
Namaste

Resources and Contacts

For information on where to find certified Yogilates classes in your area or to purchase necessary equipment such as yoga mats, blankets, blocks, and clothing, please visit

www.yogilates.com
or call toll-free 1-877-964-4528

For information on where to find authentic Pilates classes, please check your yellow pages for local studios or see the following Web sites:

www.pilates-studio.com
www.pilatesmethodalliance.org
www.themethodpilates.com

For information on where to find hatha yoga classes, please check your yellow pages for local studios or visit the following Web sites:

www.yogadirectory.com
www.yogasite.com
www.yogajournal.com
www.yimag.com

Index